DIAGNOSIS

Rare Medical Cases

VOLUME I

EVERETT MILES, M.D.

FREE REIGN

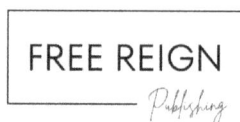

FREE REIGN
Publishing

CONTENTS

INTRODUCTION

Welcome to *Diagnosis: Rare Medical Cases*, a series that delves into the enigmatic and often perplexing world of rare medical conditions. I am Dr. Everett Miles, a practicing physician with over two decades of experience in internal medicine and diagnostics. Throughout my career, I have encountered a myriad of medical mysteries that have challenged the boundaries of my knowledge and expertise. This series aims to share these extraordinary cases with you, providing insight into the complexities and nuances of diagnosing and treating rare diseases.

Medicine is a field where every day brings new challenges, and sometimes those challenges come in the form of conditions so rare that they defy conventional medical wisdom. These cases often require not only a deep understanding of medical science but also an element of detective work, piecing together seemingly unrelated symptoms to arrive at a correct diagnosis. It is in these moments that the true art of medicine is revealed.

In each volume of this series, you will be taken on a journey through real-life cases that I have encountered in my practice. These stories are not only about the diseases themselves but also about the patients who lived through them. You will meet individuals who faced incredible odds, their courage and resilience shining through as they navigated the uncertain waters of their diagnoses. Their stories are a testament to the human spirit and the incredible advances in medical science that continue to evolve.

Each chapter will present a different case, detailing the patient's symptoms, the diagnostic process, and the eventual treatment. Along the way, I will provide insights into the medical thinking and decision-making processes that guided each case. You will gain a deeper understanding of how doctors approach complex cases and the importance of considering the rare and unusual when common diagnoses do not fit.

My hope is that this series will not only inform and educate but also inspire a greater appreciation for the intricacies of the human body and the remarkable field of medicine. Whether you are a medical professional, a student, or simply someone with a keen interest in medical science, I invite you to join me in exploring these fascinating and often bewildering medical mysteries.

Thank you for embarking on this journey with me. Together, we will uncover the stories behind some of the rarest and most intriguing medical cases ever encountered.

Dr. Everett Miles, MD

BASSEN-KORNZWEIG SYNDROME

As a pediatrician with a focus on metabolic disorders, I was well-versed in the symptoms and diagnostic processes for rare conditions. The patient, an eight-year-old child, presented to my clinic with a series of troubling symptoms. The parents reported chronic diarrhea, difficulty in gaining weight, and a noticeable decline in their child's ability to see in low light conditions. Additionally, the patient had been suffering from frequent nosebleeds and exhibited poor muscle coordination.

The patient's medical history revealed a persistent pattern of fat malabsorption since infancy, which was initially misattributed to common gastrointestinal conditions. A thorough physical examination showed that the child was markedly underweight for their age and had a distended abdomen. Palpation revealed hepatomegaly, a clear sign of liver enlargement. Additionally, the patient displayed neurological abnormalities, including diminished deep tendon reflexes and ataxia.

Given the constellation of symptoms, my differential diagnosis included conditions such as celiac disease, cystic fibrosis, and other metabolic disorders. However, the presence of night blindness, fat malabsorption, and neurological deficits pointed me towards a rarer possibility: Bassen-Kornzweig syndrome, also known as abetalipoproteinemia.

To confirm this suspicion, I ordered a series of tests. The first was a lipid profile, which revealed extremely low levels of cholesterol and triglycerides. This finding was indicative of impaired lipid transport, a hallmark of abetalipoproteinemia. Subsequently, I performed a complete blood count, which showed acanthocytosis – the presence of abnormally shaped red blood cells. This was another significant clue, as acanthocytes are commonly found in patients with this condition.

Further confirmation came from genetic testing. We conducted a molecular analysis of the MTTP gene, responsible for encoding the microsomal triglyceride transfer protein (MTP). Mutations in this gene lead to the characteristic lipid transport defects seen in abetalipoproteinemia. The results confirmed my diagnosis: the patient had a homozygous mutation in the MTTP gene.

The treatment for Bassen-Kornzweig syndrome is

multifaceted, focusing primarily on dietary management and supplementation to address the deficiencies and prevent complications. I initiated an aggressive nutritional therapy regimen tailored to the patient's specific needs.

The patient's diet was modified to include medium-chain triglycerides (MCTs) instead of long-chain triglycerides, as MCTs are absorbed directly into the bloodstream and do not require the transport mechanisms that are defective in abetalipoproteinemia. This dietary change was crucial in improving the patient's nutrient absorption.

Due to the malabsorption of fat-soluble vitamins (A, D, E, and K), high-dose vitamin supplementation was essential. Vitamin A was administered to combat the night blindness and support overall eye health. Vitamin E, which acts as a potent antioxidant, was crucial for preventing further neurological damage. Vitamin K was supplemented to help with blood clotting issues, and Vitamin D was provided to support bone health and prevent osteoporosis.

Regular follow-up visits were scheduled to monitor the patient's progress and make necessary adjustments to the treatment plan. Blood tests were conducted periodically to track lipid levels and ensure the effectiveness of the dietary modifications and vitamin supplementation. Liver function tests were also part of the routine monitoring to detect any signs of liver damage early.

Over the course of the first few months, the patient showed significant improvement. The chronic diarrhea subsided, and there was noticeable weight gain. The night blindness, although not completely resolved, showed marked improvement with the administration of Vitamin A. The neurological symptoms also stabilized; the patient's coordination improved, and the frequency of nosebleeds decreased.

However, the journey was not without challenges. Adherence to the strict dietary regimen was difficult for the patient and their family. Despite this, their commitment to the treatment plan was commendable, and the benefits were evident.

As months turned into years, the patient continued to show progress. The regular intake of MCTs and fat-soluble vitamins became a routine part of their life. School performance improved as the neurological symptoms were kept in check, and the patient was able to engage in activities previously impossible due to the lack of coordination and muscle strength.

Despite the overall positive trajectory, it was crucial to remain vigilant. Abetalipoproteinemia is a chronic condition, and the risk of complications, particularly related to the nervous system and liver, remained. Therefore, annual comprehensive evaluations were instituted to monitor for potential late-onset complications such as retinitis pigmentosa and progressive neuropathy.

Long-term management of Bassen-Kornzweig syndrome requires a sustained effort from both the medical team and the patient's family. The patient's treatment plan evolved as they grew older, transitioning from pediatric to adult care while maintaining the same principles of dietary management and supplementation.

Regular neurological assessments were critical to detect any subtle changes that might indicate the progression of the disease. Electromyography (EMG) and nerve conduction studies were periodically conducted to evaluate peripheral nerve function.

Given the risk of retinitis pigmentosa, annual visits to an ophthalmologist were necessary. These visits included comprehensive eye exams and retinal imaging to monitor for any degenerative changes.

Hepatomegaly was a persistent concern, necessitating regular liver function tests and ultrasound imaging to monitor for signs of liver disease or cirrhosis. The possibility of liver transplantation was discussed as a last resort if significant liver dysfunction developed.

Continuous monitoring of bone density was important to prevent osteoporosis, especially given the patient's increased risk due to fat malabsorption and potential vitamin D deficiency.

By the time the patient reached adulthood, they had

managed to lead a relatively normal life, albeit with the ongoing need for medical supervision and adherence to their dietary and supplementation regimen. The early diagnosis and comprehensive treatment had significantly improved their quality of life and prognosis.

While the patient did not experience a complete cure, the improvements in their health and quality of life were substantial. The careful balance of medical management and patient compliance allowed for a positive outcome in a condition that, without treatment, could have led to severe and progressive disabilities.

2

ABETALIPOPROTEINEMIA

As a physician with a specialty in gastroenterology and metabolic disorders, I have encountered numerous rare and challenging cases. One such case that remains etched in my memory is that of a patient diagnosed with Abetalipoproteinemia (ABL), a rare genetic disorder affecting lipid metabolism. This case is particularly noteworthy due to its complexity and the comprehensive approach required for diagnosis and management.

❦

THE PATIENT FIRST CAME TO MY CLINIC AT THE AGE OF 14, referred by their primary care physician due to chronic diarrhea, failure to thrive, and significant neurological symptoms including ataxia and peripheral neuropathy. Upon initial examination, the patient appeared pale, with a thin build and a notably unsteady gait. The history revealed that these symptoms had been present since early childhood but had progressively worsened over the past few years.

Given the constellation of symptoms, I suspected a metabolic or malabsorptive disorder. The initial laboratory tests included a complete blood count (CBC), liver function tests (LFTs), and a comprehensive metabolic panel. The CBC revealed mild anemia with a hemoglobin level of 10 g/dL and a mean corpuscular volume (MCV) of 90 fL, indicating normocytic anemia. LFTs showed mild elevation in transaminases. The metabolic panel was largely unremarkable except for low cholesterol levels.

To further evaluate the cause of the patient's symptoms, I ordered a more detailed lipid profile, which showed extremely low levels of total cholesterol, low-density lipoprotein (LDL), and very low-density lipoprotein (VLDL). Triglycerides were also significantly reduced. These findings were highly suggestive of a disorder affecting lipid transport or synthesis.

I then proceeded with genetic testing to confirm the diagnosis. DNA sequencing of the MTTP gene, which encodes the microsomal triglyceride transfer protein, was performed. The results revealed a homozygous mutation consistent with Abetalipoproteinemia. This confirmed the diagnosis, as the MTTP gene mutation impairs the assembly and secretion of apolipoprotein B-containing lipoproteins, leading to the characteristic lipid abnormalities seen in this condition.

Abetalipoproteinemia is an autosomal recessive disorder characterized by the absence of apolipoprotein B-containing lipoproteins, including chylomicrons, VLDL, and LDL. The mutation in the MTTP gene disrupts the normal function of the microsomal triglyceride transfer protein, which is essential for the assembly and secretion of these lipoproteins. This leads to fat malabsorption, resulting in steatorrhea and deficiency of fat-soluble vitamins (A, D, E, and K), which are critical for various bodily functions.

The neurological symptoms in ABL are primarily due to vitamin E deficiency, which is crucial for neuronal integrity and function. The patient's ataxia and peripheral neuropathy were consistent with this deficiency. Additionally, the chronic diarrhea and failure to thrive were direct consequences of fat malabsorption.

ॐ

TREATMENT OF ABETALIPOPROTEINEMIA IS multifaceted and requires a combination of dietary management and pharmacological interventions. The primary goals are to correct the nutritional deficiencies and manage the symptoms to improve the patient's quality of life.

- Dietary Management: <u>Low-Fat Diet</u>: The patient was advised to adhere to a low-fat diet to minimize steatorrhea and gastrointestinal symptoms. The diet included medium-chain triglycerides (MCTs) as they are absorbed directly into the portal circulation and do not require chylomicron formation. <u>Fat-Soluble Vitamins Supplementation</u>: High doses of fat-soluble vitamins were prescribed to address the deficiencies. Specifically, vitamin A (25,000 IU/day), vitamin D (2,000 IU/day), vitamin E (800-1,200 IU/day), and vitamin K (10 mg/week) were administered. The doses were adjusted based on regular monitoring of serum levels and clinical response.
- Pharmacological Treatment: <u>Vitamin E</u>: Given the critical role of vitamin E in neurological function, the patient was started on a high dose of vitamin E (d-alpha-tocopherol) at 800-1,200 IU/day. This was essential to prevent further neurological deterioration and potentially reverse some of the existing symptoms. <u>L-Carnitine</u>: Supplementation with L-carnitine (50-100

mg/kg/day) was also considered to support energy production and improve muscle function.

- Regular Monitoring and Follow-Up: The patient was scheduled for regular follow-up visits every three months initially, with a focus on monitoring growth parameters, neurological status, and nutritional markers. Blood tests were conducted at each visit to measure levels of fat-soluble vitamins, liver enzymes, and lipid profile to ensure adequate absorption and to adjust supplementation as needed. Neurological assessments, including nerve conduction studies and coordination tests, were performed to track the progress of neuropathy and ataxia.

Over the first six months of treatment, the patient's condition showed notable improvement. The gastrointestinal symptoms, particularly diarrhea, significantly decreased with the low-fat diet and MCT supplementation. The patient gained weight and showed improved growth parameters, indicating better nutritional status.

The most remarkable progress was observed in the neurological symptoms. After six months of high-dose vitamin E therapy, the patient's ataxia improved, and there was a marked reduction in the severity of peripheral neuropathy. The patient reported better coordination and less frequent episodes of stumbling and falling.

Despite these improvements, the patient's condition required ongoing management. Long-term adherence to the dietary regimen and vitamin supplementation was essential to maintain the benefits and prevent recurrence of symptoms. The patient and their family were educated extensively on the importance of compliance with the treatment plan and the potential complications of untreated vitamin deficiencies.

The key to long-term success lies in continuous monitoring and adjustment of treatment based on clinical and biochemical parameters.

In this case, after one year of consistent treatment and follow-up, the patient's condition stabilized. The neurological symptoms were well-controlled, and the patient demonstrated normal growth and development for their age. There were no new complications, and the patient adapted well to the dietary changes.

The patient continued to receive regular follow-up care every six months, including blood tests to monitor vitamin levels and liver function. The vitamin doses were adjusted periodically to ensure optimal levels. The patient also underwent annual neurological assessments to detect any subtle changes that might require intervention.

This case of Abetalipoproteinemia illustrates the

importance of a comprehensive and multidisciplinary approach to managing rare genetic disorders. Early diagnosis, meticulous dietary management, and targeted pharmacological therapy can significantly improve outcomes and enhance the quality of life for patients with ABL. While the condition remains a lifelong challenge, the progress observed in this patient underscores the potential for successful management with diligent care and patient compliance.

The patient in this case did not experience a complete "cure" but achieved a stable and manageable condition, which is a realistic and favorable outcome for individuals with Abetalipoproteinemia.

✣ 3 ✣

YELLOW NAIL SYNDROME

The patient, a middle-aged individual, presented with yellow discoloration of the nails, chronic cough, and swelling in the lower extremities. The yellowing of the nails was the most striking feature. The patient reported that this discoloration had been progressively worsening over the past six months. Additionally, they experienced intermittent episodes of respiratory distress and a persistent cough that did not respond to conventional treatments, such as antibiotics and bronchodilators. The lower limb swelling had also gradually developed, and it was most noticeable after prolonged standing or physical activity.

The patient's medical history was notable for chronic sinusitis and recurrent respiratory infections over the past two years. There was no significant history of smoking, exposure to environmental toxins, or family history of similar symptoms.

Upon physical examination, the patient's nails were uniformly yellow, thickened, and exhibited increased curvature with transverse ridging. The nails on both hands and feet were affected. Palpation of the lower extremities revealed pitting edema extending up to the knees. Auscultation of the lungs revealed bilateral crackles, particularly in the lower lobes, suggestive of fluid accumulation.

Given the constellation of symptoms, Yellow Nail Syndrome was suspected. To confirm the diagnosis and rule out other potential causes, a series of investigations were undertaken:

- Nail Clippings and Cultures: Nail samples were taken to rule out fungal infections. The cultures returned negative.
- Chest X-ray and High-Resolution CT Scan: The chest X-ray showed bilateral pleural effusions and signs of chronic sinusitis. The high-resolution CT scan of the chest confirmed these findings and also revealed bronchiectasis, a common respiratory manifestation in YNS.
- Pulmonary Function Tests (PFTs): PFTs demonstrated a restrictive pattern with

reduced lung volumes, consistent with the presence of pleural effusions and chronic lung disease.

- Lymphoscintigraphy: This imaging test was performed to assess the lymphatic system and confirmed lymphatic obstruction in the lower extremities, which was contributing to the lymphedema.
- Blood Tests: Complete blood count, liver function tests, renal function tests, and thyroid function tests were all within normal limits. Immunological screening was negative for autoimmune diseases.

The treatment plan for the patient focused on managing the symptoms and underlying causes associated with Yellow Nail Syndrome.

1. Respiratory Management:

- Thoracentesis: Given the significant pleural effusions, thoracentesis was performed to drain the excess fluid and alleviate respiratory distress. This procedure provided immediate symptomatic relief.
- Antibiotics: A course of broad-spectrum antibiotics was initiated to manage the recurrent respiratory infections. The patient

was closely monitored for any signs of infection, and sputum cultures were regularly obtained to guide antibiotic therapy.

- Bronchodilators and Inhaled Corticosteroids: These were prescribed to manage the bronchiectasis and reduce inflammation in the airways.
- Pulmonary Rehabilitation: The patient was enrolled in a pulmonary rehabilitation program, which included breathing exercises and physical therapy to improve lung function and overall stamina.

2. Management of Lymphedema:

- Compression Therapy: Compression stockings were prescribed to manage the lymphedema. The patient was instructed on proper usage and the importance of consistent wear to prevent fluid accumulation.
- Manual Lymphatic Drainage (MLD): Regular sessions with a certified lymphedema therapist were scheduled to facilitate lymphatic drainage and reduce swelling.
- Diuretics: Diuretics were considered but used with caution due to their limited efficacy in managing lymphedema in YNS.

3. Nail Care:

- Topical Vitamin E: Application of topical vitamin E was recommended to improve nail health and appearance. This was aimed at reducing the yellow discoloration and enhancing the strength of the nails.
- Regular Monitoring: The patient was advised to maintain regular follow-ups with a dermatologist to monitor nail changes and manage any secondary infections or complications.

The patient was followed closely over the next several months. Regular follow-up visits were scheduled to monitor the progression of symptoms and the effectiveness of the treatment plan.

- Respiratory Symptoms: The patient's respiratory symptoms showed significant improvement. The pleural effusions reduced in size, and the chronic cough became less frequent. Pulmonary function tests showed gradual improvement, indicating better lung capacity and function. The patient reported fewer respiratory infections, likely due to the combined effect of antibiotics and improved pulmonary care.

- Lymphedema: The lymphedema remained a challenge. While compression therapy and manual lymphatic drainage provided some relief, the patient continued to experience episodes of swelling, especially after physical exertion. The diuretics were not significantly effective, but the patient was educated on lifestyle modifications to manage the condition better, such as elevating the legs and avoiding prolonged standing.
- Nail Health: The yellow discoloration of the nails persisted, though there was a slight improvement in their thickness and strength with the use of topical treatments. The patient continued regular visits with the dermatologist for ongoing care.

Over the course of one year, the patient's condition stabilized. While Yellow Nail Syndrome has no definitive cure, the multidisciplinary approach to managing the symptoms allowed the patient to maintain a reasonable quality of life. The patient's respiratory function was significantly better, reducing the risk of severe infections and hospitalizations. The lymphedema was managed to a point where it did not severely impact daily activities.

The patient adapted to living with the nail changes, understanding that these were a hallmark of the syndrome but did not pose a direct health threat.

Yellow Nail Syndrome remains a rare and challenging condition to manage. While the patient did not achieve complete resolution of symptoms, the tailored management plan significantly improved their quality of life and mitigated the most debilitating aspects of the syndrome.

4

MADELUNG'S DISEASE

The patient, a 48-year-old male, presented to the clinic with complaints of progressive, painless swelling in the neck, shoulders, and upper arms. He reported that the swelling had been developing over the past two years, but he had delayed seeking medical attention because it did not cause him pain or significant discomfort initially. However, in recent months, the patient noticed the masses were becoming more pronounced, leading to difficulty in wearing clothes and mild limitations in the range of motion of his neck.

During the initial examination, I observed diffuse, symmetrical fatty deposits around the neck (giving the appearance of a "bull neck"), upper back, and upper arms. The patient's history was significant for chronic alcoholism, consuming an average of six to eight units of alcohol daily for the past twenty years. He also reported occasional numbness and tingling in his hands.

Given the clinical presentation, I considered several differential diagnoses, including lipomatosis, Cushing's syndrome, and Madelung's disease (multiple symmetric lipomatosis). I ordered a series of diagnostic tests to narrow down the possibilities:

1. Blood Tests:

- Complete blood count (CBC)
- Liver function tests (LFTs)
- Lipid profile
- Thyroid function tests
- Plasma glucose and HbA1c

2. Imaging:

- Ultrasound of the neck and upper arms
- Computed tomography (CT) scan of the neck and thorax

3. Nerve Conduction Studies:

- To evaluate the cause of the patient's numbness and tingling

The blood tests revealed elevated liver enzymes,

indicative of hepatic stress likely secondary to chronic alcohol consumption. His lipid profile showed dyslipidemia with elevated triglycerides and low high-density lipoprotein (HDL) cholesterol. Thyroid function tests were within normal limits. The nerve conduction studies indicated mild peripheral neuropathy, consistent with alcohol-related neuropathy.

Ultrasound examination demonstrated multiple, well-defined, hypoechoic masses in the subcutaneous tissue of the neck and upper arms. The CT scan provided a more detailed assessment, revealing large, symmetric adipose tissue deposits without evidence of encapsulation, consistent with multiple symmetric lipomatosis.

Based on the clinical presentation, history, and diagnostic findings, I diagnosed the patient with Madelung's disease, also known as multiple symmetric lipomatosis. This rare disorder is characterized by abnormal, symmetric fat deposition primarily in the cervical region, upper arms, and trunk, and it is often associated with chronic alcoholism and metabolic disturbances.

The treatment of Madelung's disease primarily focuses on addressing the underlying factors, managing symptoms, and improving the patient's quality of life. I discussed the following management plan with the patient:

1. Lifestyle Modifications:

- Complete cessation of alcohol consumption to prevent further progression of the disease and reduce the risk of liver damage.
- Dietary modifications to manage dyslipidemia, including a low-fat, high-fiber diet rich in fruits, vegetables, and lean proteins.
- Regular physical activity to aid weight management and improve overall health.

2. Medical Therapy:

- Medications for Dyslipidemia:

1. Atorvastatin 40 mg daily to manage elevated cholesterol levels.
2. Omega-3 fatty acid supplements to help reduce triglyceride levels.

- Neuropathy Management:

1. Gabapentin 300 mg daily for symptomatic relief of peripheral neuropathy.

- Liver Support:

1. Ursodeoxycholic acid 250 mg twice daily to support liver function.

3. <u>Surgical Intervention:</u>

- I referred the patient to a plastic surgeon for evaluation regarding liposuction or surgical excision of the fatty deposits. Surgical intervention is often considered for cosmetic reasons and to relieve mechanical discomfort or functional limitations.

I scheduled the patient for follow-up appointments at three-month intervals to monitor his progress and response to treatment. During each visit, we reassessed his adherence to lifestyle modifications, medication effectiveness, and any new or persisting symptoms.

At the first follow-up, the patient reported significant efforts to reduce his alcohol intake, though he had not completely abstained. His lipid profile showed modest improvements, but liver enzymes remained elevated. The patient was encouraged to continue working towards complete alcohol cessation and adherence to dietary recommendations.

Six months into the treatment plan, the patient had successfully reduced his alcohol consumption to minimal levels and demonstrated good adherence to his medication regimen. His lipid profile showed further improvement, and liver enzymes began to normalize. However, the fatty deposits remained prominent and continued to cause mechanical discomfort and social distress.

The patient underwent a thorough evaluation by a plastic surgeon, who recommended a combination of liposuction and direct excision to remove the larger adipose deposits. The surgery was performed in stages to minimize complications and allow for better aesthetic outcomes.

The surgical interventions were successful in significantly reducing the size of the fatty deposits, particularly around the neck and shoulders. The patient reported considerable relief from the mechanical discomfort and improved mobility. The cosmetic results were satisfactory, greatly enhancing the patient's self-esteem and social interactions.

Post-surgery, the patient was closely monitored for any signs of recurrence, which is a known possibility with Madelung's disease. He continued on his medication regimen and maintained lifestyle modifications. Regular follow-up appointments included physical examinations, lipid profile assessments, and liver function tests to ensure ongoing management of his condition.

Over the next two years, the patient remained free from significant recurrence of the fatty deposits. He achieved complete abstinence from alcohol, which was a critical factor in preventing disease progression and supporting liver health. His lipid profile and liver function tests normalized, indicating a positive response to the combined lifestyle and medical interventions.

Despite the chronic nature of Madelung's disease, the patient's adherence to the treatment plan resulted in a stable and manageable condition. Regular monitoring and prompt intervention at any sign of recurrence remained essential components of his long-term care.

While the condition posed significant physical and social challenges, comprehensive management led to substantial improvements in his quality of life.

5

BALANTIDIASIS

The patient, a middle-aged man, presented to the clinic with severe abdominal pain, chronic diarrhea, and a notable loss of weight. He had been experiencing these symptoms for approximately two weeks. His stool was occasionally tinged with blood, and he reported frequent episodes of nausea and vomiting. Upon initial assessment, the patient appeared dehydrated and malnourished. He had been working in a rural area with poor sanitation, a detail that would later prove significant.

The patient's medical history was unremarkable. He had no known chronic conditions, allergies, or significant past surgeries. On physical examination, his abdomen was tender to palpation, especially in the lower quadrants. There were no signs of peritonitis, but hyperactive bowel sounds were present, indicating increased intestinal activity. His vital signs showed tachycardia, hypotension, and a low-grade fever.

Given the symptoms and the patient's history, I decided to order a series of diagnostic tests to determine the cause of his condition. Blood tests revealed leukocytosis, indicative of an infection or inflammatory process. His electrolyte levels were deranged, with hypokalemia and hyponatremia, likely due to prolonged diarrhea.

Stool samples were sent for microbiological analysis, including bacterial culture, ova, and parasite examination, as well as molecular tests for enteric pathogens. An abdominal ultrasound was performed, which showed diffuse bowel wall thickening but no abscesses or free fluid in the peritoneum.

The stool examination was pivotal in diagnosing the patient. Microscopic analysis revealed the presence of large ciliated protozoa, identified as *Balantidium coli*. This organism is the causative agent of balantidiasis, an infection predominantly associated with swine and contaminated water sources. Given the patient's history of working in a rural area with poor sanitation, it became clear that he had likely contracted the infection through fecal-oral transmission.

Balantidium coli is a large, motile protozoan that can colonize the human large intestine, particularly the cecum and colon. It has a trophozoite form, which is ciliated and motile, and a cyst form, which is resistant and can survive outside the host. The trophozoites invade the intestinal mucosa, causing ulceration, which explains the patient's abdominal pain, diarrhea, and occasional bloody stools. The organism's presence induces an inflammatory response, leading to the observed leukocytosis and fever.

Treatment of balantidiasis involves both addressing the infection and managing the patient's symptoms and dehydration. I initiated the following treatment plan:

- Antibiotic Therapy: The patient was prescribed tetracycline, 500 mg four times daily for ten days. Tetracycline is the drug of choice for balantidiasis due to its efficacy in eradicating *Balantidium coli*. For patients intolerant to tetracycline, metronidazole or iodoquinol could be used as alternatives.
- Hydration and Electrolyte Management: The patient received intravenous fluids to correct his dehydration and electrolyte imbalances. Normal saline with potassium supplementation was administered to address his hypokalemia.
- Symptomatic Treatment: To manage his nausea and vomiting, antiemetic medication (ondansetron) was prescribed. For pain relief, a combination of acetaminophen and an

antispasmodic (hyoscine butylbromide) was used.

- Nutritional Support: Given his malnourished state, the patient was started on a high-calorie, high-protein diet. Initially, he was given nutritional support through oral supplements and later through regular meals as his condition improved.

The patient was admitted to the hospital for close monitoring due to the severity of his symptoms and the need for intravenous therapy. Over the next few days, his diarrhea began to subside, and his abdominal pain decreased. Repeat stool examinations were performed on the fourth and tenth days of treatment to monitor the eradication of the parasite. By the end of the antibiotic course, no Balantidium coli trophozoites or cysts were detected in his stool samples.

After ten days of treatment, the patient showed significant improvement. His diarrhea had resolved, his abdominal pain was minimal, and he had regained some weight. His electrolyte levels normalized, and he was able to maintain hydration with oral intake alone. He was discharged from the hospital with instructions to continue a balanced diet and maintain good hygiene practices to prevent reinfection.

At the time of discharge, I provided the patient with

detailed education on the importance of proper sanitation and hygiene, especially given his occupation. He was advised to ensure safe drinking water and avoid contact with contaminated sources. Regular follow-up appointments were scheduled to monitor his recovery and ensure there were no relapses.

The patient's long-term prognosis was favorable. Balantidiasis, when promptly diagnosed and appropriately treated, typically resolves without long-term complications. However, the patient was warned about the potential for recurrence, particularly if he returned to the same environmental conditions that led to his initial infection.

Balantidiasis, although rare in developed countries, remains a significant health issue in areas with inadequate sanitation. Early diagnosis and treatment are crucial in preventing complications and ensuring patient recovery.

6

WARM AUTOIMMUNE HEMOLYTIC ANEMIA

I remember the patient vividly. It was a Monday morning, and the hospital was bustling as usual. The patient was a middle-aged individual who had come to the emergency department complaining of fatigue, shortness of breath, and jaundice. As I reviewed their case, I noted the significant pallor and yellowish tint to their skin, which immediately raised my suspicion of a hemolytic process.

The initial laboratory tests were revealing. The patient's hemoglobin level was alarmingly low at 7.0 g/dL, and their reticulocyte count was elevated, indicating increased red blood cell (RBC) production by the bone marrow in response to anemia. Their lactate dehydrogenase (LDH) levels were elevated, and haptoglobin levels were undetectable, all pointing towards hemolysis. The peripheral blood smear showed spherocytes, which are

RBCs that appear spherical rather than the usual biconcave shape, suggesting an autoimmune etiology.

To confirm my suspicion, I ordered a direct antiglobulin test (DAT), also known as the direct Coombs test. The DAT was positive for IgG antibodies and complement (C3), solidifying the diagnosis of Warm Autoimmune Hemolytic Anemia (WAIHA). WAIHA is an autoimmune disorder where the body produces antibodies that mistakenly target and destroy its own RBCs at body temperature. This condition can lead to severe anemia and is often associated with other autoimmune diseases, lymphoproliferative disorders, or infections.

The treatment plan for WAIHA is multi-faceted, focusing on stopping the immune system from attacking RBCs, managing symptoms, and addressing any underlying causes. I started the patient on corticosteroids, the first-line treatment for WAIHA. Prednisone was prescribed at a high dose of 1 mg/kg/day. Corticosteroids work by suppressing the immune response, thus reducing the production of antibodies against RBCs.

While the patient was being treated with steroids, I also initiated supportive care. This included transfusions of packed RBCs to manage the severe anemia. However, transfusions in WAIHA can be tricky due to the presence of autoantibodies, which can complicate the cross-matching process. We had to ensure that the transfused blood was as compatible as possible by performing extended cross-matching and using RBCs that lacked the antigens to which the patient's antibodies were directed.

In addition to corticosteroids and transfusions, I prescribed folic acid supplements. Hemolysis increases the demand for folate due to the high turnover of RBCs, and folic acid supplementation helps support the increased erythropoiesis in the bone marrow.

As I monitored the patient's response to treatment, it became clear that while there was some improvement, it was not as robust as I had hoped. The hemoglobin levels stabilized but remained low, and the patient continued to exhibit signs of hemolysis. Given the partial response to corticosteroids, I decided to introduce a second-line treatment: rituximab.

Rituximab is a monoclonal antibody that targets CD20, a protein found on the surface of B cells. By depleting B cells, rituximab reduces the production of autoantibodies. The patient received rituximab at a dose of 375 mg/m^2 once weekly for four weeks. Rituximab has shown efficacy in patients with WAIHA who are refractory to corticosteroids or who require steroid-sparing agents.

Throughout the treatment, I closely monitored the patient's progress with regular blood tests, including complete blood counts (CBC), reticulocyte counts, and levels of LDH and haptoglobin. It was a delicate balance to manage the side effects of immunosuppression while ensuring adequate control of hemolysis.

Over the next few weeks, the patient began to show significant improvement. The hemoglobin levels gradually increased, and the markers of hemolysis, such as LDH and bilirubin, decreased. The patient's energy levels improved, and the jaundice resolved. By the end of the rituximab course, the hemoglobin had normalized, and the DAT showed a reduction in autoantibody levels.

In addition to medical management, I explored potential underlying causes of the patient's WAIHA. A thorough workup included screening for infections, autoimmune diseases, and malignancies. Tests for common infections such as Epstein-Barr virus (EBV), cytomegalovirus (CMV), and Mycoplasma pneumoniae were negative. Screening for autoimmune diseases, including systemic lupus erythematosus (SLE), rheumatoid arthritis, and thyroid disorders, also yielded no significant findings. Imaging studies and bone marrow biopsy were performed to rule out lymphoproliferative disorders, and fortunately, these were unremarkable.

After several months of treatment and follow-up, the patient remained in remission. The prednisone was gradually tapered and eventually discontinued, and the patient remained off steroids without relapse. Rituximab had provided a durable response, and the patient's quality of life had significantly improved.

However, I emphasized the importance of regular follow-up and monitoring. WAIHA can be a chronic condition with potential for relapse, and it was crucial to detect and manage any recurrence early. The patient was advised to seek immediate medical attention if they noticed any signs of anemia or hemolysis, such as fatigue, jaundice, or dark urine.

In summary, managing WAIHA required a comprehensive approach involving corticosteroids, immunosuppressive therapy with rituximab, and supportive care. The key to successful treatment was careful monitoring and adjusting the therapy based on the patient's response.

The patient eventually regained their health and returned to their daily activities.

7

ABLEPHARON-MACROSTOMIA SYNDROME

The patient, a neonate, was born at full term following an uneventful pregnancy. The labor and delivery were unremarkable, and the patient was delivered via spontaneous vaginal delivery. The initial Apgar scores were 8 and 9 at one and five minutes, respectively. Upon physical examination shortly after birth, several congenital anomalies were noted, prompting further evaluation.

Upon initial inspection, the patient exhibited several distinct features. The most striking were the absence of eyelids (ablepharon), an unusually wide mouth (macrostomia), and malformed ears. Additionally, there were sparse scalp hair and eyebrows, redundant skin, and syndactyly of fingers and toes.

Given the constellation of these anomalies, a clinical suspicion of Ablepharon-Macrostomia Syndrome (AMS) was raised. AMS is a rare genetic disorder characterized by the congenital absence of eyelids, wide mouth, ear anomalies, and various other craniofacial, digital, and cutaneous abnormalities.

To confirm the diagnosis and assess the extent of the associated anomalies, a series of diagnostic tests were ordered:

1. Genetic Testing: A comprehensive genetic panel was performed to identify any mutations in the TWIST2 gene, which is known to be associated with AMS.

2. Ophthalmologic Examination: Detailed examination to evaluate the severity of the ablepharon and potential damage to the corneal surface due to exposure.

3. Audiometric Testing: Hearing tests to determine if the ear malformations were associated with hearing loss.

4. Imaging Studies: Cranial and abdominal ultrasonography to detect any internal anomalies, such as renal or cardiac defects, commonly associated with AMS.

5. Dermatologic Consultation: Evaluation of the skin condition, including assessment of skin redundancy and potential interventions.

Genetic testing revealed a heterozygous mutation in

the TWIST2 gene, confirming the clinical diagnosis of Ablepharon-Macrostomia Syndrome. This mutation is typically inherited in an autosomal dominant pattern, although de novo mutations are also possible.

Given the complexity of the condition, a multidisciplinary approach was essential for the patient's management. The following specialties were involved:

1. Pediatric Surgery: For the correction of craniofacial anomalies.

2. Ophthalmology: For the management of ablepharon and protection of the cornea.

3. Otolaryngology: For the evaluation and treatment of ear anomalies and hearing loss.

4. Dermatology: For the management of skin abnormalities.

5. Genetic Counseling: To provide information and support to the family regarding the genetic nature of the condition and implications for future pregnancies.

The first priority was the protection of the corneal surface due to the absence of eyelids. The patient underwent an emergency tarsorrhaphy, a procedure where the eyelids are partially sewn together to protect the cornea from exposure. This was followed by staged reconstructive surgeries to create functional eyelids using local skin flaps and grafts.

The macrostomia was addressed through surgical procedures aimed at reducing the size of the mouth and reshaping the lips. This involved careful planning to ensure functional and aesthetic outcomes. Multiple staged surgeries were performed to gradually reduce the mouth size and improve the alignment of the lips.

The malformed ears required surgical correction to improve both the appearance and potentially the function, although the initial hearing tests indicated that the patient had some degree of conductive hearing loss. Reconstructive surgery of the ears was performed, followed by fitting of hearing aids to improve auditory function.

The redundant skin was managed through excision and skin tightening procedures. This was performed in stages to minimize the risk of complications and ensure proper healing. The patient also received treatments to promote hair growth and manage the sparse hair condition.

The postoperative period was critical for the patient's recovery. The patient was monitored closely for any signs of infection, particularly in the areas of surgical intervention. Pain management was also a priority, with appropriate analgesics administered to ensure comfort.

Regular follow-up visits were scheduled with all involved specialties to monitor the progress of healing and plan further interventions as needed. The patient underwent physical and occupational therapy to support overall development and improve fine motor skills affected by the syndactyly.

The long-term management of the patient involved ongoing monitoring and support. Despite the complex nature of the condition, the multidisciplinary approach ensured that the patient received comprehensive care.

The reconstructed eyelids functioned well, and the corneal surface remained healthy with regular lubrication and protective measures. Vision development was closely monitored, and any refractive errors were corrected with glasses.

Hearing tests were performed regularly to assess the effectiveness of the hearing aids and any changes in auditory function. Speech therapy was also provided to support language development.

The patient continued to receive care from craniofacial and dermatologic specialists to address any residual or new issues. Regular skin checks and interventions were performed to manage the redundant skin and hair growth.

The family received ongoing support and education about the genetic aspects of AMS. This included discussions about the risk of recurrence in future pregnancies and the availability of prenatal testing.

The prognosis for patients with Ablepharon-Macrostomia Syndrome varies depending on the severity of the anomalies and the effectiveness of the interventions. In this case, the patient showed significant improvement with the multidisciplinary approach. The surgical corrections provided functional and aesthetic benefits, and the supportive therapies contributed to overall development.

The patient continued to face challenges, particularly in terms of ongoing medical care and potential psychosocial impacts. However, the comprehensive management plan ensured that these challenges were addressed proactively.

Ablepharon-Macrostomia Syndrome is a rare and complex genetic disorder requiring a coordinated, multidisciplinary approach for effective management. In this case, early diagnosis and timely surgical interventions were crucial in addressing the congenital anomalies and improving the patient's quality of life.

While the patient will require ongoing medical care and support, the collaborative efforts of the healthcare team have laid a strong foundation for continued progress. This case underscores the importance of a holistic approach in managing rare congenital conditions and highlights the potential for positive outcomes with appropriate medical and surgical interventions.

8

DIPETALONEMIASIS

The patient, a middle-aged man from a rural area, presented with a set of symptoms that had progressively worsened over several months. He initially reported experiencing generalized weakness, malaise, and intermittent fevers. Upon further questioning, he mentioned episodes of pruritus, especially at night, and a sense of discomfort in his lower extremities. These symptoms raised my suspicion of a possible parasitic infection, given his living conditions and lack of recent travel history.

Physical examination revealed significant findings: generalized lymphadenopathy, particularly in the inguinal and axillary regions, along with a mildly enlarged spleen. Additionally, I noted numerous small, non-tender nodules under the skin, predominantly on his limbs and trunk. These observations, coupled with his symptoma-tology, pointed towards a potential filarial infection.

To confirm the diagnosis, I ordered a complete blood count, which showed eosinophilia with an absolute eosinophil count significantly above normal levels. This was a strong indicator of a parasitic infection. Given the suspicion of a filarial infection, I proceeded with a peripheral blood smear, stained with Giemsa, taken at night when microfilariae are most active in the peripheral blood.

The blood smear examination under microscopy revealed microfilariae characteristic of the genus Dipetalonema. These microfilariae were sheathed and displayed a distinct pattern of nuclei, helping differen-tiate them from other filarial species. To further confirm the diagnosis, I sent a blood sample for PCR testing, which identified the DNA of Dipetalonema spp., solidi-fying the diagnosis of dipetalonemiasis.

With the diagnosis confirmed, the next step was to devise an appropriate treatment plan. Dipetalonemiasis, being a filarial infection, requires a multi-faceted approach to effectively eliminate both adult worms and microfilariae.

1. Ivermectin: This drug is effective against microfilar-iae. I prescribed a single oral dose of 200 µg/kg. Iver-

mectin works by binding to glutamate-gated chloride channels, increasing the permeability of the cell membrane to chloride ions, leading to paralysis and death of the microfilariae.

2. Doxycycline: To target the endosymbiotic Wolbachia bacteria, which are essential for the survival of adult filarial worms, I prescribed doxycycline at a dose of 200 mg daily for six weeks. The bacterium's eradication not only affects the fertility of the adult worms but also leads to their death over time.

3. Albendazole: This broad-spectrum anthelmintic was included to target adult worms. I prescribed 400 mg twice daily for three weeks. Albendazole works by inhibiting the polymerization of tubulin into micro-tubules, disrupting essential cellular processes in the parasite.

4. Antihistamines and Corticosteroids: Given the potential for an intense immune response leading to Mazzotti reaction (severe inflammatory response due to dying microfilariae), I prescribed antihistamines and a short course of corticosteroids to mitigate these effects.

The patient was admitted for initial observation to monitor for adverse reactions to the medications, particularly the risk of a Mazzotti reaction. Within the first 24 hours of starting ivermectin, he experienced mild itching and a low-grade fever, which were managed with antihistamines and antipyretics. There were no severe reactions, and he was discharged with detailed instructions to return for regular follow-ups.

Over the next few weeks, the patient reported a gradual improvement in his symptoms. The pruritus and nodular lesions began to diminish, and his energy levels improved. Regular blood tests showed a decreasing trend in eosinophil counts, indicative of a successful response to the treatment.

After completing the course of doxycycline and albendazole, a follow-up blood smear was performed. The peripheral blood smear showed a significant reduction in the number of microfilariae, and PCR testing was negative for Dipetalonema DNA. The patient's clinical symptoms had substantially improved, with no further episodes of fever or generalized weakness.

A final follow-up six months post-treatment showed no recurrence of symptoms, and repeated blood tests confirmed the absence of microfilariae. The patient was considered to have been successfully treated for dipetalonemiasis.

This case of dipetalonemiasis highlights the importance of considering parasitic infections in patients with nonspecific systemic symptoms, particularly in endemic areas. Early diagnosis and a comprehensive treatment plan targeting both the microfilariae and adult worms, as well as their symbiotic bacteria, are crucial for successful management. The patient's recovery underscores the effectiveness of a combination therapy approach, providing a roadmap for future cases of filarial infections.

9

HEREDITARY CERULOPLASMIN DEFICIENCY

The patient, a 32-year-old male, came to the clinic with complaints of worsening tremors, unsteady gait, and slurred speech over the past year. He had noticed these symptoms progressively impairing his daily activities, making it difficult for him to perform tasks that required fine motor skills. The patient also reported chronic fatigue and had a history of mild anemia for several years, which had been treated with iron supplements without significant improvement.

The patient's family history was notable for neurological and liver issues. His father had been diagnosed with Wilson's disease and had passed away at the age of 45 due to liver failure. However, the patient's own serum copper and urinary copper levels were within normal ranges, ruling out Wilson's disease. His mother had no significant medical history, and there was no known history of similar symptoms in siblings or other relatives.

During the physical examination, the patient exhibited several noteworthy findings. His skin had a bronze discoloration, particularly noticeable on his face and hands. Neurological examination revealed dysarthria (slurred speech), ataxia (lack of muscle coordination), and dystonia (involuntary muscle contractions). The patient's liver was palpable and slightly enlarged, suggesting hepatomegaly. Given the combination of these symptoms and the patient's family history, I decided to conduct a series of specialized tests.

The initial workup included a complete blood count (CBC), liver function tests (LFTs), serum ceruloplasmin level, and imaging studies. The CBC revealed microcytic anemia with hemoglobin levels at 10.5 g/dL (normal range: 13.8-17.2 g/dL) and mean corpuscular volume (MCV) of 70 fL (normal range: 80-100 fL). Liver function tests showed elevated transaminases: alanine transaminase (ALT) at 85 U/L (normal range: 7-56 U/L) and aspartate transaminase (AST) at 90 U/L (normal range: 10-40 U/L), indicating liver dysfunction.

The critical finding was the serum ceruloplasmin level, which was significantly low at 3 mg/dL (normal range: 20-40 mg/dL). This suggested a defect in ceruloplasmin production or function. To confirm the diagnosis, I ordered genetic testing for mutations in the CP gene, which encodes ceruloplasmin. Meanwhile, magnetic resonance imaging (MRI) of the brain was performed to assess iron deposition.

The MRI revealed hyperintensities in the basal ganglia, indicating iron accumulation. Genetic testing confirmed a homozygous mutation in the CP gene, consistent with hereditary ceruloplasmin deficiency, also known as aceruloplasminemia. This rare autosomal recessive disorder results in the absence or dysfunction of ceruloplasmin, a protein essential for iron and copper metabolism.

Hereditary ceruloplasmin deficiency is characterized by the absence or malfunction of ceruloplasmin, a ferroxidase enzyme that oxidizes Fe^{2+} to Fe^{3+}. This oxidation is necessary for iron binding to transferrin and subsequent transport to various tissues. Without functional ceruloplasmin, iron accumulates in tissues, particularly in the liver, pancreas, and brain, leading to oxidative stress and cellular damage.

The patient's neurological symptoms were attributed to iron deposition in the basal ganglia, which is critical for motor control. Iron overload in the liver led to hepatomegaly and elevated liver enzymes, while iron accumulation in the skin caused the observed bronze discoloration. The microcytic anemia was due to disrupted iron metabolism and ineffective erythropoiesis.

The primary treatment goal for hereditary ceruloplasmin deficiency is to reduce iron overload and manage symptoms. I initiated iron chelation therapy with defer-oxamine, an iron chelator that binds free iron and promotes its excretion. Deferoxamine was administered via subcutaneous infusion using a portable pump for 8-12 hours daily. The patient was instructed on the proper use of the pump and advised to adhere strictly to the infusion schedule to maximize the efficacy of the treatment.

In addition to deferoxamine, I prescribed oral zinc acetate at a dose of 50 mg three times daily. Zinc acetate helps reduce gastrointestinal iron absorption by inducing the production of metallothionein in enterocytes, which binds dietary iron and prevents its entry into the bloodstream.

Given the patient's neurological symptoms, I referred him to a neurologist for further evaluation and symptomatic management. The neurologist prescribed medications to alleviate tremors and dystonia, and recommended physical therapy to improve coordination and mobility. The patient was also advised to follow a diet low in iron and to avoid iron supplements and foods high in iron.

Regular monitoring was essential to assess the effectiveness of the treatment and to adjust dosages as needed. I scheduled monthly follow-ups to evaluate the patient's clinical status, iron levels, and liver function. Blood tests, including serum ferritin and transferrin saturation, were performed to monitor iron stores. Liver function tests were repeated to track liver enzyme levels.

MRI scans of the brain were scheduled every six months to monitor iron deposition. The neurologist also conducted regular assessments to evaluate the patient's neurological symptoms and adjust medications accordingly.

Over the first three months of treatment, the patient's serum ferritin levels decreased significantly, indicating a reduction in iron stores. His liver enzyme levels also improved, with ALT and AST decreasing to 60 U/L and 55 U/L, respectively. Clinically, the patient reported feeling less fatigued and noticed an improvement in his tremors and coordination. His skin discoloration became less pronounced, and his overall quality of life improved.

Despite the initial success of the treatment, the patient developed complications related to long-term iron chelation therapy. After two years, he reported symptoms of mild hearing loss and blurred vision. Audiometric tests confirmed sensorineural hearing loss, and an ophthalmologic examination revealed retinal changes, both of which are known side effects of prolonged deferoxamine use.

To mitigate these side effects, I reduced the dosage and frequency of deferoxamine and introduced deferasirox, an oral iron chelator, as an alternative.

Deferasirox was started at a dose of 20 mg/kg once daily, with close monitoring for any adverse effects. This change in treatment helped alleviate the side effects while maintaining control over iron levels.

Despite adjustments in treatment, the patient's neurological condition gradually declined over the next few years. MRI scans continued to show persistent iron deposition in the basal ganglia, and his neurological symptoms became more pronounced. He developed progressive dementia, severe motor impairment, and required assistance with daily activities. The neurologist prescribed additional medications to manage these symptoms and recommended continued physical and occupational therapy.

The patient also developed signs of liver cirrhosis, including ascites and jaundice. Liver function tests showed worsening liver enzymes and evidence of synthetic dysfunction, such as low albumin levels and prolonged prothrombin time. A liver biopsy confirmed cirrhosis, and the patient was referred to a hepatologist for further management. The hepatologist considered the possibility of liver transplantation but deemed the patient a high-risk candidate due to his deteriorating neurological status and overall health.

Despite aggressive management, the patient's condition continued to worsen. He experienced recurrent infections due to immunosuppression from liver dysfunction and iron overload. These infections further compromised his health, leading to multiple hospitalizations.

At the age of 38, the patient succumbed to complications related to iron overload and liver cirrhosis. An autopsy revealed extensive iron deposition in the liver, pancreas, and brain, consistent with hereditary ceruloplasmin deficiency. The liver showed advanced cirrhosis with nodular regeneration, and the brain exhibited severe iron accumulation in the basal ganglia and cerebellum.

Hereditary ceruloplasmin deficiency is a rare genetic disorder with significant clinical challenges. The absence of ceruloplasmin disrupts iron metabolism, leading to multi-organ damage. The combination of neurological symptoms, liver dysfunction, and iron overload requires a high index of suspicion and a thorough diagnostic workup.

Early diagnosis and prompt initiation of iron chelation therapy are crucial to prevent irreversible damage. However, long-term chelation therapy carries the risk of significant side effects, necessitating careful monitoring and adjustments in treatment. The use of alternative chelators, such as deferasirox, can help mitigate these risks but requires close follow-up.

This case highlights the importance of a multidisciplinary approach in managing hereditary ceruloplasmin deficiency. Collaboration between neurologists, hepatologists, hematologists, and other specialists is essential to address the complex needs of these patients. Supportive therapies, including physical and occupational therapy, play a critical role in improving the quality of life for patients with neurological impairments.

Ongoing research is needed to develop more effective treatments with fewer side effects. Gene therapy holds promise as a potential cure for hereditary ceruloplasmin deficiency by restoring normal ceruloplasmin production. Advances in our understanding of iron metabolism and the role of ceruloplasmin may lead to new therapeutic targets and strategies.

In the meantime, raising awareness about this rare disorder among healthcare providers is essential to ensure timely diagnosis and management. Genetic counseling should be offered to affected families to discuss the risk of transmission and reproductive options.

Hereditary ceruloplasmin deficiency is a rare and challenging disorder with significant implications for patients. Early recognition and aggressive management can improve outcomes, but the progressive nature of the disease often leads to substantial morbidity and mortality. This case underscores the need for continued research and development of targeted therapies to better address the challenges posed by this rare genetic disorder.

10

MEGAESOPHAGUS

When I first saw the patient, his chief complaints were consistent with severe dysphagia and regurgitation. These symptoms are hallmark presentations of esophageal motility disorders. Dysphagia, the sensation of difficulty swallowing, can be classified as either oropharyngeal or esophageal. The patient's history suggested esophageal dysphagia, given the sensation of food getting stuck in the lower chest area.

The patient's presentation led me to suspect achalasia, an esophageal motility disorder characterized by the failure of the LES to relax and the absence of esophageal peristalsis. The pathophysiology of achalasia involves the degeneration of the myenteric plexus, particularly affecting the inhibitory neurons responsible for the relaxation of the LES. The exact etiology remains unclear, but it is thought to involve autoimmune mechanisms, viral infections, or genetic predispositions.

To confirm the diagnosis, I ordered a barium swallow study. This radiographic examination involves the patient swallowing barium sulfate, a contrast medium, which then coats the lining of the esophagus and allows for detailed X-ray imaging. The classic finding of a "bird-beak" appearance at the gastroesophageal junction, along with a dilated esophagus, was evident in our patient. This appearance results from the narrowed LES and the dilated proximal esophagus due to retained food and secretions.

Next, an esophagogastroduodenoscopy (EGD) was performed. EGD allows direct visualization of the esophageal mucosa and can rule out other potential causes of dysphagia, such as malignancies, strictures, or eosinophilic esophagitis. In this patient, the EGD confirmed a markedly dilated esophagus with retained food particles but no obstructive lesions or mucosal abnormalities.

The definitive diagnostic test for achalasia is esophageal manometry. This test measures the pressure dynamics within the esophagus and LES. Our patient's manometry findings showed an elevated resting pressure of the LES, incomplete relaxation of the LES during swallowing, and aperistalsis in the esophageal body. These findings are diagnostic of type II achalasia, characterized by pan-esophageal pressurization and preserved residual pressure at the LES.

Once the diagnosis was confirmed, we discussed various treatment options with the patient. The primary aim of treatment in achalasia is to reduce LES pressure to facilitate esophageal emptying and relieve symptoms. Treatment options include:

1. Pneumatic Dilation: This involves endoscopic insertion of a balloon that is inflated to disrupt the LES muscle fibers. It is effective but carries a risk of esophageal perforation.

2. Surgical Myotomy: The Heller myotomy involves cutting the LES muscle fibers to reduce pressure. It can be performed laparoscopically and is often combined with a fundoplication to prevent reflux.

3. Pharmacologic Therapy: Medications such as nitrates or calcium channel blockers can temporarily reduce LES pressure but are often not sufficient for severe cases.

4. Botulinum Toxin Injection: Endoscopic injection of botulinum toxin into the LES can temporarily reduce LES pressure but requires repeated treatments and is generally reserved for patients who are not surgical candidates.

Given the patient's relatively good health and the

severity of his symptoms, we opted for a laparoscopic Heller myotomy with partial fundoplication. This approach offered a high success rate and long-term symptom relief.

The patient underwent preoperative assessments to ensure he could tolerate the procedure. These assessments included complete blood counts, metabolic panels, chest X-ray, and ECG. All results were within normal limits, and he was cleared for surgery.

The laparoscopic Heller myotomy was performed under general anesthesia. The procedure involved five small abdominal incisions through which a laparoscope and surgical instruments were inserted. The esophagus was carefully mobilized, and the muscle fibers of the LES were cut longitudinally, extending onto the gastric cardia. This myotomy effectively reduced the LES pressure, allowing easier passage of food into the stomach.

To prevent postoperative gastroesophageal reflux, a partial fundoplication (Dor fundoplication) was performed. This involves wrapping the fundus of the stomach around the posterior aspect of the esophagus to create a valve mechanism that reduces the risk of reflux.

The surgery was completed without complications. The patient was transferred to the recovery unit for postoperative monitoring. His vital signs remained stable, and he showed steady improvement. He was initially kept on a clear liquid diet and gradually advanced to a soft diet over the following days. His symptoms of dysphagia and regurgitation resolved remarkably, and he began to regain weight.

The patient was discharged on postoperative day five with instructions to follow a modified diet and avoid strenuous activities for several weeks. At his two-week follow-up appointment, he reported significant improvement in his quality of life. He had no difficulty swallowing, and his nutritional status was improving.

A repeat barium swallow study confirmed a patent gastroesophageal junction with good passage of contrast into the stomach, indicating successful myotomy. Over the next six months, the patient continued to do well. He adhered to dietary modifications and followed up regularly to monitor for potential complications, such as GERD.

Postoperative complications of Heller myotomy can include gastroesophageal reflux, esophageal perforation, and persistent dysphagia. Our patient developed mild gastroesophageal reflux, managed with proton pump inhibitors (PPIs). He was advised on lifestyle modifications, such as elevating the head of the bed, avoiding late meals, and limiting foods that trigger reflux.

At each follow-up visit, we monitored his progress and adjusted his treatment as needed. His weight steadily increased, and his nutritional status normalized. He experienced occasional mild chest discomfort, which we attributed to esophageal spasms and managed with calcium channel blockers. These symptoms gradually resolved over time.

The long-term prognosis for patients with achalasia treated with Heller myotomy is generally favorable. Most patients experience significant symptom relief and improved quality of life. However, long-term follow-up is essential to monitor for potential complications, such as the development of esophageal carcinoma, which has a higher incidence in patients with long-standing achalasia.

Our patient's outcome was positive. At his one-year follow-up, he remained symptom-free, with no recurrence of dysphagia or regurgitation. His nutritional status was excellent, and he had regained his pre-illness weight. Surveillance endoscopy performed at one year showed no evidence of mucosal abnormalities or Barrett's esophagus, a condition that can develop due to chronic gastroesophageal reflux.

This case of megaesophagus secondary to achalasia highlights the importance of early diagnosis and timely intervention. Achalasia, although rare, should be considered in patients presenting with progressive dysphagia and regurgitation. A thorough diagnostic approach, including barium swallow, EGD, and esophageal manometry, is essential for accurate diagnosis and classification.

The treatment of achalasia aims to relieve the obstruction at the LES and improve esophageal emptying. Laparoscopic Heller myotomy with partial fundoplication is a highly effective treatment option with durable results. Postoperative follow-up is crucial to monitor for complications and ensure long-term success.

This patient's case underscores the importance of a multidisciplinary approach involving gastroenterologists, surgeons, and dietitians to achieve optimal outcomes. Through careful evaluation, appropriate intervention, and ongoing management, patients with achalasia can achieve significant symptom relief and improved quality of life.

Reflecting on this case, I am reminded of the complexities of managing esophageal motility disorders and the critical role of individualized patient care. Each patient presents unique challenges and requires a tailored approach to achieve the best possible outcomes. This case serves as a valuable learning experience and reinforces the importance of vigilance and thoroughness in medical practice.

🦋 11 🦋

DIABETIC BEARDED WOMAN SYNDROME

The patient, a 58-year-old female, presented to the clinic with several distressing symptoms. She reported an increase in facial hair growth, specifically on her chin and upper lip, which she found particularly embarrassing and socially debilitating. Additionally, she complained of profound fatigue, frequent urination (polyuria), and unintentional weight loss amounting to approximately 15 pounds over the past six months. Her medical history was significant for type 2 diabetes mellitus, diagnosed ten years prior, and poorly controlled due to sporadic medication adherence and irregular follow-up visits.

Upon physical examination, the patient exhibited notable hirsutism. Her blood pressure was elevated at 150/95 mmHg, and she had a body mass index (BMI) of 32 kg/m², classifying her as obese. Her skin showed signs of acanthosis nigricans, characterized by dark, velvety patches, particularly around the neck and underarms, indicative of severe insulin resistance. Additionally, she had multiple skin tags around her neck.

Given the combination of her symptoms and physical findings, my differential diagnosis included poorly controlled type 2 diabetes with possible polycystic ovary syndrome (PCOS) or an adrenal disorder such as Cushing's syndrome or an androgen-secreting tumor. I ordered a comprehensive panel of laboratory tests, including fasting blood glucose, HbA1c, serum electrolytes, liver function tests, renal function tests, and a complete blood count. Furthermore, I requested specific tests for hyperandrogenism, including serum testosterone, dehydroepiandrosterone sulfate (DHEA-S), and a 24-hour urinary free cortisol level to evaluate potential adrenal dysfunction.

The laboratory results were revealing and included the following:

- Fasting blood glucose: 220 mg/dL (normal: <100 mg/dL)
    - HbA1c: 9.8% (normal: <5.7%)
    - Serum electrolytes: within normal limits
    - Liver function tests: mildly elevated AST and ALT
    - Renal function tests: normal
    - Complete blood count: normal

Of particular note were the hormonal levels:

- Elevated serum testosterone: 78 ng/dL (normal for females: 15-70 ng/dL)

   - Elevated DHEA-S: 500 µg/dL (normal for females: 65-380 µg/dL)

   - Normal 24-hour urinary free cortisol levels, ruling out Cushing's syndrome

The elevated serum testosterone and DHEA-S levels, combined with the clinical presentation, confirmed the diagnosis of Diabetic Bearded Woman Syndrome (DBWS), a rare condition characterized by hirsutism and hyperandrogenism in the context of poorly controlled diabetes.

Diabetic Bearded Woman Syndrome is an uncommon but well-documented phenomenon in which women with poorly controlled diabetes develop hyperandrogenism. The pathophysiology involves insulin resistance, a hallmark of type 2 diabetes, leading to compensatory hyperinsulinemia. High insulin levels can directly stimulate the ovaries to produce more androgens. Additionally, insulin decreases the hepatic production of sex hormone-binding globulin (SHBG), which increases the availability of free testosterone in the blood. The result is a clinical picture of hirsutism, androgenic alopecia, and other signs of hyperandrogenism.

In this patient, the chronic hyperglycemia and insulin resistance likely exacerbated the androgen excess, leading to her pronounced symptoms. Her clinical features were typical of DBWS, with significant facial hirsutism, acanthosis nigricans, and the metabolic complications of poorly controlled diabetes.

The primary goals of treatment were to achieve stringent glycemic control and address the hyperandrogenism. I developed a multifaceted treatment approach, encompassing pharmacologic therapy, lifestyle modifications, and supportive measures:

1. Glycemic Control:

  - Initiated a basal-bolus insulin regimen. The patient started on long-acting insulin glargine at bedtime and rapid-acting insulin lispro before meals. The goal was to achieve preprandial glucose levels of 80-130 mg/dL and postprandial levels below 180 mg/dL.

  - Emphasized the importance of consistent medication adherence and regular monitoring of blood glucose levels. Provided education on the use of a glucometer and the significance of maintaining a blood glucose diary.

2. Lifestyle Modifications:

  - Referred the patient to a registered dietitian for a personalized meal plan focusing on low glycemic index foods, portion control, and weight reduction. The dietitian provided strategies to incorporate healthy eating habits into her daily routine.

- Recommended a gradual increase in physical activity, starting with 30 minutes of moderate exercise, such as walking, most days of the week. The goal was to improve insulin sensitivity, promote weight loss, and enhance overall cardiovascular health.

3. Pharmacologic Management of Hyperandrogenism:

- Prescribed spironolactone, an anti-androgen, at a dose of 50 mg twice daily. Spironolactone acts as an androgen receptor antagonist and inhibits androgen production, helping to reduce hirsutism.

- Initiated metformin at 500 mg twice daily. Metformin, in addition to its glucose-lowering effects, has been shown to reduce hyperandrogenism in women with PCOS-like symptoms. It helps improve insulin sensitivity and may aid in weight reduction.

4. Adjunctive Therapies:

- Discussed the option of cosmetic treatments for facial hair, such as laser hair removal or electrolysis, to be considered once her diabetes was better controlled. These treatments would help improve her self-esteem and quality of life.

- Provided psychological support and counseling to address the emotional and social impact of her condition. Referred her to a support group for women with similar experiences, recognizing the importance of mental health in chronic disease management.

The patient was scheduled for follow-up appointments every four weeks to monitor her response to treatment, assess glycemic control, and adjust medications as necessary. During these visits, we measured fasting blood glucose, HbA1c, serum testosterone, and DHEA-S levels. Additionally, I monitored for potential side effects of the medications, such as hyperkalemia from spironolactone and gastrointestinal disturbances from metformin.

At the first follow-up visit, the patient reported adherence to the insulin regimen and dietary changes. Her fasting blood glucose had improved to 150 mg/dL, and she had lost 5 pounds. Serum testosterone and DHEA-S levels had begun to decrease, but hirsutism remained a concern. Encouraged by her progress, I reinforced the importance of continued adherence to the treatment plan and adjusted her insulin doses based on her glucose diary.

By the third follow-up, three months into the treatment, her HbA1c had dropped to 7.5%, and fasting blood glucose averaged 120 mg/dL. She experienced a significant reduction in hirsutism, with less facial hair requiring removal. However, she developed mild hyperkalemia, a known side effect of spironolactone, necessitating a dose adjustment to 25 mg twice daily. I also addressed her concerns about occasional hypoglycemic episodes by adjusting her insulin doses and providing education on recognizing and managing hypoglycemia.

Six months into the treatment, the patient presented with mild pedal edema and complained of persistent fatigue. Laboratory tests revealed normal renal function but elevated liver enzymes (AST and ALT). Suspecting a possible drug-induced liver injury from metformin or spironolactone, I temporarily discontinued both medications and substituted metformin with pioglitazone, a thiazolidinedione, to maintain glycemic control. I closely monitored liver enzymes, which gradually normalized over the next few weeks. The patient's glycemic control remained stable with the new regimen, and her HbA1c dropped further to 6.8%.

One year after the initial presentation, the patient's diabetes was well-controlled, with an HbA1c of 6.5% and fasting blood glucose consistently below 130 mg/dL. Her serum testosterone and DHEA-S levels were within normal ranges, and she reported significant improvement in hirsutism, managed with periodic laser hair removal sessions. Despite initial challenges, the patient demonstrated remarkable adherence to her treatment plan and lifestyle modifications. She experienced substantial weight loss, improved physical fitness, and enhanced overall well-being.

Throughout the treatment period, the patient

encountered several complications requiring adjustments to her management plan:

- Hyperkalemia: The initial dose of spironolactone caused mild hyperkalemia, necessitating dose reduction and closer monitoring of serum potassium levels. I advised the patient to avoid potassium-rich foods and informed her about the signs and symptoms of hyperkalemia.

- Hypoglycemia: The patient experienced occasional hypoglycemic episodes, particularly after exercise or skipping meals. We adjusted her insulin regimen and provided additional education on carbohydrate counting, meal planning, and the importance of regular food intake.

- Drug-Induced Liver Injury: Elevated liver enzymes prompted the temporary discontinuation of metformin and spironolactone. Substituting metformin with pioglitazone proved effective in maintaining glycemic control without further liver enzyme elevation.

Long-term management of Diabetic Bearded Woman Syndrome requires a multidisciplinary approach and ongoing patient education. Key components of the patient's long-term management included:

- Continued Glycemic Control: Maintaining tight glycemic control was crucial in preventing complications and reducing hyperandrogenism. The patient continued with the basal-bolus insulin regimen, supplemented with pioglitaz one.

- Regular Monitoring: Regular follow-up visits every three to six months allowed for monitoring of blood glucose, HbA1c, serum testosterone, and DHEA-S levels. Periodic liver function tests and renal function assessments were also necessary.

- Lifestyle Modifications: The patient adhered to a healthy diet and regular physical activity, which contributed to weight loss and improved insulin sensitivity. She received ongoing support from a dietitian and participated in a diabetes management program.

- Cosmetic and Psychological Support: Periodic laser hair removal sessions helped manage hirsutism and improve the patient's self-esteem. She also benefited from psychological support and counseling to address the emotional impact of her condition.

The patient's journey underscored the importance of a holistic and patient-centered approach in managing complex endocrine disorders. Through regular follow-up, personalized treatment adjustments, and multidisciplinary support, we achieved significant clinical improvement and quality of life enhancement for the patient.

In conclusion, Diabetic Bearded Woman Syndrome, though rare, presents a unique challenge requiring a comprehensive and individualized treatment strategy. The patient's successful outcome highlights the importance of stringent glycemic control, addressing hyperandrogenism, and providing ongoing support to manage both the physical and psychological aspects of the condition. Through dedicated efforts and collaboration, we were able to transform a challenging clinical scenario into a story of recovery and resilience.

ACHONDROGENESIS

I remember the day the patient was brought to my clinic. The mother was in her second trimester of pregnancy, visibly anxious, and accompanied by her partner. They had been referred to me, a specialist in pediatric genetics, due to abnormal ultrasound findings. The initial scan had shown severe skeletal abnormalities, and the referring obstetrician suspected a rare genetic disorder. As I reviewed the images, I noted the severe shortening of the limbs, the disproportionately large head, and the narrow chest. These findings were consistent with a lethal form of skeletal dysplasia, Achondrogenesis.

Achondrogenesis is a rare and severe form of skeletal dysplasia, characterized by a failure of bone formation, leading to significant abnormalities in the development of the skeletal system. The condition is classified into three main types: Achondrogenesis type IA (Houston-Harris type), Achondrogenesis type IB (Fraccaro type), and Achondrogenesis type II (Langer-Saldino type). Each type has distinct genetic and clinical features, but all result in severe, often lethal, outcomes.

The diagnosis of Achondrogenesis was suspected based on the ultrasound findings, but definitive diagnosis required further genetic testing. I recommended an amniocentesis to obtain fetal cells for genetic analysis. The parents agreed, and the procedure was performed the following day. The sample was sent to our genetic laboratory for analysis, where we performed karyotyping and targeted genetic testing for known mutations associated with Achondrogenesis.

As we waited for the results, I explained to the parents the nature of the condition. Achondrogenesis is caused by mutations in genes involved in the development of cartilage and bone. In Achondrogenesis type IA, mutations occur in the TRIP11 gene, which encodes a protein essential for the proper function of the Golgi apparatus, a cellular structure critical for protein processing and transport. Achondrogenesis type IB is caused by mutations in the SLC26A2 gene, which encodes a sulfate transporter essential for cartilage formation. Achondrogenesis type II is caused by mutations in the COL2A1 gene, which encodes type II collagen, a major component of cartilage.

The genetic results came back within two weeks. The patient had a mutation in the SLC26A2 gene, confirming a diagnosis of Achondrogenesis type IB. This form of the disease is inherited in an autosomal recessive manner, meaning that both parents must carry one copy of the mutated gene. The parents were devastated by the news, and I spent a considerable amount of time discussing the implications and possible outcomes with them.

Achondrogenesis type IB is characterized by extreme micromelia (shortening of the limbs), a narrow thorax, and a prominent abdomen. The vertebral bodies are also severely affected, leading to a lack of normal spinal development. The prognosis for infants with Achondrogenesis type IB is poor, with most affected individuals dying in utero or shortly after birth due to respiratory failure caused by the small thoracic cavity and underdeveloped lungs.

Given the severity of the condition and the poor prognosis, the options for management were limited. I explained to the parents that there was no cure for Achondrogenesis and that treatment would be primarily supportive. They could choose to continue the pregnancy and prepare for palliative care after birth, or they could consider termination of the pregnancy. This was an incredibly difficult decision for them, and I provided as much support and information as possible to help them make an informed choice.

The parents decided to continue the pregnancy and prepare for palliative care. We arranged for a multidisciplinary team to be involved in the care of the patient after birth, including neonatologists, palliative care specialists, and genetic counselors. Our goal was to provide the best possible comfort and quality of life for the patient, however brief that life might be.

The remainder of the pregnancy was closely monitored with frequent ultrasounds to assess fetal growth and development. As expected, the skeletal abnormalities became more pronounced over time, and the growth of the thorax remained severely restricted. The parents attended counseling sessions to help them cope with the emotional burden and to prepare for the birth and subsequent care of their child.

At 36 weeks of gestation, the mother went into labor. The delivery was planned to take place in our specialized neonatal unit, where the necessary medical support would be immediately available. The patient was born via cesarean section, weighing just over two kilograms. The characteristic features of Achondrogenesis type IB were evident at birth: extremely short limbs, a narrow chest, a large head with a prominent forehead, and a distended abdomen. The skin appeared loose and wrinkled due to the lack of underlying bone structure.

The neonatology team was on hand to provide immediate care. Despite the severe skeletal abnormalities, the patient showed some signs of life, with a weak cry and minimal movement. We provided supportive care, including gentle ventilation to assist with breathing, but we knew that the patient's respiratory function was severely compromised due to the underdeveloped lungs and narrow chest cavity.

The parents were able to hold their child, and we focused on ensuring that the patient was as comfortable as possible. Pain management was a priority, and we administered analgesics to alleviate any discomfort. The palliative care team provided emotional support to the parents, helping them to create precious memories during the brief time they had with their child.

Despite our best efforts, the patient's condition deteriorated rapidly. The respiratory distress worsened, and within a few hours, the patient passed away peacefully in the arms of the parents. It was a heartbreaking moment, but I was grateful that we had been able to provide compassionate care and support to the family during this incredibly difficult time.

In the aftermath, we conducted a thorough review of the case. The genetic confirmation of Achondrogenesis type IB provided valuable information for the family and for our understanding of this rare condition. We discussed the importance of genetic counseling for the parents, as they had a 25% chance of having another child with the same condition in future pregnancies. We also reviewed the options for prenatal diagnosis in future pregnancies, including early ultrasound screening and genetic testing.

The case of the patient with Achondrogenesis type IB highlighted the challenges and complexities of managing rare genetic disorders. It underscored the importance of a multidisciplinary approach to care, involving geneticists, neonatologists, palliative care specialists, and counselors to provide comprehensive support to affected families. While there was no cure for Achondrogenesis, the goal was to provide the best possible care and to support the family through their journey.

Reflecting on the case, I was reminded of the importance of empathy and communication in the practice of medicine. Providing clear, accurate information and supporting families through difficult decisions is as crucial as the medical management itself. This case reinforced my commitment to providing compassionate, patient-centered care, particularly in the face of devastating diagnoses like Achondrogenesis.

In conclusion, the patient with Achondrogenesis type IB did not survive beyond a few hours after birth, as expected given the severity of the condition. The genetic diagnosis provided clarity and allowed for informed decision-making and planning for palliative care. The parents received comprehensive support from our multidisciplinary team, ensuring that their child's brief life was as comfortable as possible. The experience highlighted the critical role of genetic counseling and the importance of empathy and communication in managing rare and severe genetic disorders.

✣ 13 ✣
ACUTE CHOLECYSTITIS

The patient in the emergency department, presenting with severe right upper quadrant abdominal pain radiating to the back and right shoulder. The patient, a middle-aged individual, had been experiencing intermittent episodes of pain for the past few months, but this episode was markedly different in intensity and duration. Accompanying the pain were nausea, vomiting, and fever. The patient's medical history included hypertension and hyperlipidemia but no previous surgeries or significant gastrointestinal issues.

On physical examination, the patient was in obvious distress, clutching the right side of the abdomen. Vital signs revealed a fever of 38.9°C, a heart rate of 110 beats per minute, blood pressure of 145/90 mmHg, and respiratory rate of 22 breaths per minute. The patient appeared jaundiced, and the abdomen was tender to palpation in the right upper quadrant with positive Murphy's sign, indicating severe pain upon deep inspiration when palpating the gallbladder area. These findings suggested acute cholecystitis, an inflammation of the gallbladder, often due to obstruction by gallstones.

Laboratory tests were ordered, including a complete blood count (CBC), liver function tests (LFTs), pancreatic enzymes, and a comprehensive metabolic panel. The CBC showed leukocytosis with a white blood cell count of 16,000/mm^3, indicating an inflammatory response or infection. LFTs revealed elevated levels of alkaline phosphatase, aspartate aminotransferase (AST), and alanine aminotransferase (ALT), which pointed towards biliary obstruction or inflammation. Bilirubin levels were also elevated, consistent with the patient's jaundice.

An abdominal ultrasound was performed as the next step in diagnostic imaging. The ultrasound showed a thickened gallbladder wall (>3 mm), pericholecystic fluid, and a sonographic Murphy's sign, which is a sharp increase in pain when the ultrasound probe compresses the gallbladder. Gallstones were visible within the gallbladder, and there was no evidence of common bile duct stones, which ruled out choledocholithiasis. These findings confirmed the diagnosis of acute calculous cholecystitis.

Given the severity of the patient's condition, I initiated intravenous fluid resuscitation and administered broad-spectrum antibiotics to cover common biliary pathogens, including Escherichia coli, Klebsiella species, and Enterococcus. The chosen regimen was piperacillin-tazobactam, given the patient's lack of penicillin allergy and the need for comprehensive coverage. Pain management was also crucial; intravenous opioids were used judiciously to control the severe pain.

Surgical consultation was obtained promptly, as cholecystectomy, the surgical removal of the gallbladder, is the definitive treatment for acute cholecystitis. The timing of surgery is critical in these cases; early cholecystectomy within 72 hours of symptom onset is associated with better outcomes and lower complication rates compared to delayed surgery. The patient was prepared for surgery with preoperative fasting and continued intravenous fluids and antibiotics.

The patient underwent laparoscopic cholecystectomy, a minimally invasive procedure that typically involves several small incisions through which a camera and surgical instruments are inserted. During the operation, the gallbladder was found to be acutely inflamed and distended, with thickened walls and evidence of pericholecystic fluid. The cystic duct and artery were identified, clipped, and divided, and the gallbladder was carefully dissected from the liver bed and removed. The procedure was completed without intraoperative complications, and the patient was transferred to the recovery room in stable condition.

Postoperatively, the patient was monitored closely for signs of complications such as bile duct injury, bleeding, or infection. Pain control was managed with intravenous opioids initially, transitioning to oral analgesics as the patient improved. Antibiotic therapy was continued for 24 hours post-surgery to ensure adequate coverage and then discontinued. The patient's recovery was uneventful, with a gradual return to a regular diet and mobilization.

Laboratory tests repeated postoperatively showed normalization of white blood cell count and liver function tests, indicating resolution of the inflammatory process. The patient's jaundice improved, and by the time of discharge, the patient was afebrile and comfortable, with significantly reduced pain. The patient was discharged home with instructions for wound care, activity restrictions, and follow-up appointments.

In follow-up visits, the patient reported significant improvement in symptoms, with no recurrence of abdominal pain or gastrointestinal issues. The surgical wounds healed well, and there were no signs of infection or other complications. The patient was advised on lifestyle modifications, including dietary changes to reduce fat intake, given the absence of a gallbladder, which plays a role in fat digestion. The patient was also counseled on weight management and control of hyperlipidemia to prevent future biliary issues.

Acute cholecystitis typically arises due to gallstone impaction in the cystic duct, leading to increased intra-gallbladder pressure, distension, and compromised blood flow. This sets off an inflammatory cascade involving both mechanical and chemical factors, with secondary bacterial infection contributing to the inflammatory process. Diagnosis relies heavily on clinical presentation and imaging studies, with ultrasound being the gold standard due to its high sensitivity and specificity for detecting gallstones and signs of inflammation.

Management principles focus on stabilizing the patient, addressing infection and inflammation, and resolving the underlying obstruction. Early surgical intervention remains the cornerstone of treatment, with laparoscopic cholecystectomy preferred due to its minimally invasive nature, shorter recovery time, and reduced postoperative pain compared to open surgery. In certain cases where surgery is contraindicated or delayed, alternative treatments such as percutaneous cholecystostomy may be considered, though these are typically reserved for high-risk patients.

The successful outcome in this case was largely due to the prompt recognition of symptoms, appropriate use of diagnostic tools, and timely surgical intervention. The patient's adherence to postoperative care and lifestyle modifications also played a crucial role in recovery and prevention of future biliary complications.

In conclusion, this case of acute cholecystitis highlights the critical importance of a multidisciplinary approach in managing acute surgical conditions. Early diagnosis, effective medical and surgical treatment, and comprehensive postoperative care are essential in ensuring positive outcomes for patients with this common yet potentially serious condition. The patient's journey from acute illness to recovery exemplifies the effectiveness of modern medical and surgical practices in addressing acute cholecystitis.

❧ 14 ❧

SWEDISH PORPHYRIA

I had been practicing medicine for over twenty years when I encountered one of the most perplexing and challenging cases of my career: a patient with Swedish Porphyria. It began one ordinary day in my clinic when the patient, a middle-aged individual, presented with a myriad of symptoms that did not immediately point to a single diagnosis.

The patient complained of severe abdominal pain, recurrent nausea, and vomiting, symptoms that had been persisting for several weeks. Initial examinations revealed that the patient's skin had notable photosensitivity, characterized by blisters and lesions on areas exposed to sunlight. There was also a distinctive reddish-brown discoloration of the urine. These clinical manifestations were diverse and suggested multiple potential diagnoses, but none were immediately conclusive.

My first course of action was to conduct a detailed history and physical examination. The patient reported a family history of similar symptoms in several relatives, which raised the possibility of a hereditary condition. Given the broad spectrum of symptoms and the family history, I decided to run a series of laboratory tests.

I ordered blood, urine, and stool tests, focusing on the porphyrin levels, given the distinctive urine discoloration and photosensitivity. The initial tests revealed significantly elevated levels of porphyrins in the patient's urine, which was a critical clue. Porphyrins are precursors in the heme synthesis pathway, and their accumulation often points to a disorder within this pathway.

Given these results, I narrowed the differential diagnosis to a type of porphyria. Porphyrias are a group of rare inherited disorders characterized by an abnormal accumulation of porphyrin precursors due to a deficiency of specific enzymes in the heme biosynthetic pathway. The next step was to identify which type of porphyria the patient had.

To further pinpoint the diagnosis, I performed a quantitative analysis of porphyrins and porphyrin precursors in the blood and urine. The patient's results showed elevated levels of delta-aminolevulinic acid (ALA) and porphobilinogen (PBG), which are typical markers of acute porphyria. However, given the photosensitivity, I considered the possibility of a combination of acute and cutaneous porphyria.

To confirm the diagnosis, I ordered genetic testing to look for mutations in the genes associated with various types of porphyria. The results revealed a mutation in the HMBS gene, confirming a diagnosis of acute inter-mittent porphyria (AIP), specifically Swedish Porphyria. This form is particularly prevalent in Sweden and is char-acterized by a partial deficiency of the hydroxymethylbi-lane synthase enzyme.

With the diagnosis confirmed, the next step was to initiate treatment. The treatment of acute intermittent porphyria involves managing acute attacks and preventing future episodes. Acute attacks are often precipitated by factors such as certain medications, hormonal changes, and dietary influences. Therefore, I needed to identify and eliminate any potential triggers for the patient.

Firstly, I reviewed the patient's medication history and identified any drugs known to exacerbate porphyria. These included barbiturates, sulfonamide antibiotics, and certain anticonvulsants. The patient was instructed to discontinue any unsafe medications and was provided with a list of safe alternatives.

In managing the acute attack, I focused on symp-tomatic treatment and reducing the accumulation of porphyrin precursors. The patient was admitted to the hospital for close monitoring and administration of intra-venous glucose. Glucose can help by suppressing the synthesis of ALA synthase, the first enzyme in the heme pathway, thereby reducing the production of porphyrin precursors.

In addition to glucose administration, the patient received intravenous hemin, a synthetic form of heme, which acts as a negative feedback inhibitor of ALA synthase. This treatment is highly effective in reducing the levels of ALA and PBG, thereby alleviating the symp-toms of the acute attack.

The patient also required pain management, as the abdominal pain was severe and debilitating. I prescribed opioid analgesics to manage the pain, along with anti-emetic medications to control nausea and vomiting. Throughout the hospital stay, the patient was monitored for any signs of complications such as electrolyte imbal-ances or neuropathy, which can occur in severe cases of porphyria.

Over the course of several days, the patient's symp-toms gradually improved with treatment. The abdominal pain subsided, nausea and vomiting were controlled, and the skin lesions began to heal. After about a week of hospitalization, the patient was stable enough to be discharged with a detailed plan for ongoing management and prevention of future attacks.

Upon discharge, I emphasized the importance of

avoiding known triggers and maintaining a balanced diet. The patient was advised to follow a high-carbohydrate diet, as this can help suppress the synthesis of porphyrin precursors. Regular follow-up appointments were scheduled to monitor the patient's condition and adjust the treatment plan as needed.

During follow-up visits, I continued to monitor the patient's porphyrin levels through regular blood and urine tests. These tests were crucial in detecting any early signs of an impending attack and adjusting the treatment accordingly. The patient was also provided with an emergency treatment plan, including a supply of intravenous glucose and hemin, to manage any acute attacks promptly.

Over the next several months, the patient remained stable with no recurrent attacks. The photosensitivity gradually decreased, and the skin lesions healed completely. Genetic counseling was provided to the patient and their family to discuss the hereditary nature of the condition and the implications for other family members. This was particularly important given the familial history of similar symptoms.

Throughout this period, I worked closely with a team of specialists, including a geneticist, a dermatologist, and a pain management expert, to ensure comprehensive care for the patient. The geneticist provided insights into the hereditary aspects of the condition and helped guide the genetic counseling sessions. The dermatologist assisted in managing the skin lesions and advised on sun protection strategies to prevent photosensitivity-related complications. The pain management expert helped optimize the pain relief regimen, ensuring the patient could lead a comfortable life without reliance on potentially harmful medications.

One aspect of managing porphyria is educating the patient about lifestyle modifications. The patient was advised to avoid fasting and low-carbohydrate diets, as these can trigger acute attacks by increasing the demand for gluconeogenesis, thus enhancing the production of ALA and PBG. Instead, frequent small meals rich in carbohydrates were recommended. Alcohol and smoking were strictly discouraged due to their potential to precipitate attacks.

In addition to dietary management, the patient was instructed to avoid exposure to sunlight as much as possible. The use of protective clothing, broad-spectrum sunscreens, and physical barriers like hats and sunglasses were emphasized. The patient was also advised to monitor any new symptoms closely and report them immediately to prevent the progression of an acute attack.

Another critical aspect of long-term management was the psychological support for the patient. Living with a chronic condition like porphyria can be mentally taxing, and I referred the patient to a counselor to help cope with the stress and anxiety associated with the disease. Support groups for individuals with porphyria were also recommended, as they can provide a sense of community and shared experiences, which can be incredibly beneficial for mental health.

The treatment plan also included regular liver function tests, as porphyria can sometimes lead to liver complications. Monitoring liver enzymes helped ensure that any potential liver issues were detected early and managed promptly. Given the potential risk of liver damage associated with repeated hemin administration, this was an important preventive measure.

During one follow-up visit, the patient reported experiencing mild abdominal discomfort and darkening of the urine. Immediate urine tests confirmed a slight increase in porphyrin levels, indicating the early stages of an acute attack. This early detection allowed for prompt intervention with intravenous glucose and a short course of hemin, effectively preventing a full-blown attack and minimizing the patient's discomfort.

This case highlighted the importance of patient education and regular monitoring in managing chronic conditions like porphyria. By understanding the triggers and early signs of an attack, the patient was able to take proactive steps to manage the condition, leading to a significant improvement in quality of life.

Over the next few years, the patient had occasional mild flare-ups, but these were managed effectively with the established treatment plan. The patient's overall health improved, and they were able to engage in most daily activities without significant limitations. The patient also became an advocate for porphyria awareness, sharing their experience and educating others about the condition, which helped them cope with the challenges of living with a rare disease.

In summary, the diagnosis and treatment of Swedish Porphyria in this patient involved a systematic approach to identifying the underlying genetic mutation, managing acute symptoms, and preventing future attacks. The key to successful management was early recognition of the condition, prompt treatment with glucose and hemin, and ongoing monitoring to prevent recurrences. The patient responded well to treatment and was able to return to a normal, active life with appropriate lifestyle modifications and medical management.

❧ 15 ❧

PRIMARY ADRENAL INSUFFICIENCY

As a physician with years of experience, I have encountered many challenging cases, but one of the most memorable involved a patient with primary adrenal insufficiency, also known as Addison's disease. This condition, characterized by the failure of the adrenal glands to produce adequate amounts of hormones, presented a complex clinical picture that required careful diagnostic work and meticulous management.

The patient first presented to my clinic with complaints of severe fatigue, muscle weakness, and significant weight loss over several months. These symptoms, while non-specific, were progressively worsening and had started to impact their daily activities significantly. During the initial physical examination, I noted notable hyperpigmentation of the skin, particularly in sun-exposed areas and in the creases of the hands, elbows, and knuckles. This clinical sign was particularly telling and immediately raised my suspicion of Addison's disease, given its association with chronic adrenal insufficiency.

To confirm my clinical suspicion, I ordered a comprehensive panel of laboratory tests. The initial serum cortisol measurement was strikingly low, particularly given the time of day the blood was drawn (early morning when cortisol levels should be highest). Concurrently, the plasma adrenocorticotropic hormone (ACTH) level was significantly elevated. This combination of low cortisol and high ACTH strongly suggested a primary adrenal insufficiency, as the elevated ACTH indicated the pituitary gland was functioning correctly and attempting to stimulate the adrenal glands without success.

Additionally, the patient's basic metabolic panel revealed hyponatremia (low sodium levels) and hyperkalemia (elevated potassium levels). These electrolyte disturbances are hallmark features of Addison's disease due to the lack of aldosterone, which normally helps to regulate sodium and potassium balance. The patient's serum sodium was markedly low at 125 mmol/L (normal range: 135-145 mmol/L), and potassium was elevated at 5.8 mmol/L (normal range: 3.5-5.0 mmol/L).

To further confirm the diagnosis, I proceeded with an ACTH stimulation test. This involves administering synthetic ACTH (cosyntropin) and measuring the serum cortisol response at intervals post-injection. In a healthy individual, cortisol levels would rise significantly following ACTH administration. In this patient's case, the cortisol levels showed minimal increase, further confirming the diagnosis of primary adrenal insufficiency.

Having confirmed Addison's disease, the next step was to identify the underlying etiology. Autoimmune adrenalitis is the most common cause of primary adrenal insufficiency in developed countries. To explore this possibility, I ordered tests for adrenal autoantibodies, specifically 21-hydroxylase antibodies, which came back positive. This confirmed that the patient's adrenal insufficiency was due to autoimmune destruction of the adrenal cortex.

With the diagnosis firmly established, immediate treatment was imperative. The cornerstone of treatment for Addison's disease is hormone replacement therapy to replace the deficient adrenal hormones. I initiated the patient on hydrocortisone to replace cortisol and fludrocortisone to replace aldosterone. Hydrocortisone was prescribed in a regimen that aimed to mimic the body's natural diurnal rhythm of cortisol secretion, with the largest dose administered in the morning and a smaller dose in the afternoon. This approach helps to manage symptoms and maintain physiological cortisol levels throughout the day.

Fludrocortisone was prescribed once daily to address the aldosterone deficiency, and the dose was carefully adjusted based on the patient's blood pressure, serum electrolytes, and clinical response. In addition to pharmacotherapy, comprehensive patient education was essential. I explained the critical importance of strict adherence to the medication regimen, the need to recognize early signs of adrenal crisis, and the requirement for dose adjustments during periods of stress, illness, or surgery. The patient was also provided with an emergency injection kit containing hydrocortisone to be used in case of an adrenal crisis, a potentially life-threatening condition characterized by severe hypotension, dehydration, and shock.

The patient's initial response to treatment was promising. Over the next few weeks, there was a noticeable improvement in their symptoms. The profound fatigue lessened, muscle strength began to return, and their weight stabilized. Follow-up appointments were scheduled at regular intervals to monitor the patient's clinical progress and adjust medication doses as necessary. During these visits, I paid close attention to their blood pressure, serum electrolytes, and overall well-being.

However, managing Addison's disease is fraught with challenges. Despite initial improvements, the patient experienced an adrenal crisis several months into treatment. They presented to the emergency department with symptoms of severe weakness, confusion, abdominal pain, and profound hypotension. Recognizing the urgency of the situation, immediate resuscitation was initiated. Intravenous fluids were administered to address dehydration and hypotension, and high-dose intravenous hydrocortisone was given to rapidly replace the deficient cortisol. The patient's condition stabilized after a few hours, underscoring the critical importance of rapid recognition and treatment of adrenal crisis.

Following recovery from the adrenal crisis, a detailed review of the patient's management plan was conducted to identify potential gaps. It became evident that the patient had not appropriately increased their hydrocortisone dose during a recent gastrointestinal illness, which likely precipitated the crisis. This incident highlighted the need for reinforced education on the importance of stress dosing and meticulous management during intercurrent illnesses.

Given the complexity of long-term management of Addison's disease, I referred the patient to an endocrinologist for specialized care. The endocrinologist conducted a thorough evaluation and made adjustments to the hormone replacement regimen to optimize the patient's quality of life. This included exploring options for modified-release hydrocortisone formulations, which can provide more stable cortisol levels throughout the day, potentially reducing the risk of adrenal crises.

Throughout this journey, the patient remained compliant with their treatment and proactive in managing their condition. They wore a medical alert bracelet indicating their diagnosis of Addison's disease and carried an emergency card detailing their condition and treatment plan. Despite the challenges, the patient's condition remained stable with no further episodes of adrenal crisis. Regular follow-ups and laboratory tests ensured that their hormone levels were adequately replaced, and their quality of life was maintained. The patient's resilience and adherence to treatment played a pivotal role in their positive outcome.

Reflecting on this case, it underscores the importance of early recognition, accurate diagnosis, and comprehensive management of primary adrenal insufficiency. Addison's disease, while rare, can have significant morbidity and mortality if not properly treated. It requires a multidisciplinary approach involving primary care physicians, endocrinologists, and patient education to ensure optimal outcomes. The patient's journey also highlights the potential complications and the need for vigilance in managing intercurrent illnesses to prevent adrenal crises. Through continued education, support, and regular monitoring, patients with Addison's disease can lead healthy and fulfilling lives.

This case remains a testament to the complexity of endocrine disorders and the critical role of hormone replacement therapy in restoring normal physiology. It also emphasizes the importance of patient empowerment and education in managing chronic conditions. The patient's successful management of primary adrenal insufficiency serves as a reminder of the profound impact of timely and appropriate medical intervention.

One notable aspect of Addison's disease management involves the careful monitoring and adjustment of medication doses. For hydrocortisone, the goal is to use the lowest effective dose to minimize potential side effects, such as osteoporosis, weight gain, and glucose intolerance. Regular bone density scans and monitoring for signs of metabolic syndrome are important aspects of ongoing care. Fludrocortisone dosing is adjusted based on blood pressure readings and serum electrolyte levels, particularly sodium and potassium.

In addition to pharmacologic therapy, lifestyle modifications play a crucial role in the management of Addison's disease. Patients are advised to maintain a balanced diet with adequate salt intake, particularly in the context of aldosterone deficiency, which can lead to sodium loss. Regular exercise, stress management techniques, and adequate hydration are also important to maintain overall health and prevent complications.

Periodic re-evaluation by an endocrinologist ensures

that the treatment regimen remains appropriate as the patient ages or as new health issues arise. Advances in medical technology, such as continuous subcutaneous hydrocortisone infusion pumps, are being explored as potential options for more precise hormone replacement. Research into the genetics and pathophysiology of autoimmune adrenalitis may also lead to novel therapeutic approaches in the future.

Patient education is a cornerstone of managing chronic conditions like Addison's disease. Patients must understand the importance of medication adherence, recognize early symptoms of adrenal insufficiency, and know how to respond in emergencies. Support groups and counseling can provide additional resources and emotional support for patients and their families.

In conclusion, the management of primary adrenal insufficiency, or Addison's disease, is multifaceted and requires a comprehensive approach involving accurate diagnosis, appropriate hormone replacement therapy, patient education, and regular follow-up care. The case of this patient illustrates the challenges and rewards of managing a complex endocrine disorder. Through diligent medical care and patient cooperation, individuals with Addison's disease can achieve stability and maintain a good quality of life. This experience has reinforced my commitment to providing thorough, compassionate care to all patients facing chronic medical conditions.

❧ 16 ❧

CRIBRIFORM CARCINOMA

As a practicing oncologist, I've encountered numerous malignancies, but the case of cribriform carcinoma presented unique challenges that pushed the boundaries of my medical expertise. This particular patient's journey, from diagnosis through treatment to eventual outcome, exemplified the complexities and demands of oncology.

The patient, a 52-year-old individual, presented with a palpable lump in the left breast. Initial physical examination suggested a possible malignancy. A mammogram was performed, revealing an irregular mass with spiculated margins, a classic radiographic indication of breast cancer. An ultrasound followed, which confirmed the presence of a 2.5 cm hypoechoic lesion with irregular borders. Given these findings, a core needle biopsy was deemed necessary for definitive diagnosis.

The biopsy samples were sent for histopathological examination. The pathologist reported the presence of atypical cells arranged in cribriform patterns, characteristic of cribriform carcinoma. Cribriform carcinoma is a rare subtype of invasive ductal carcinoma, accounting for about 0.8-3.5% of all breast cancers. The hallmark of this malignancy is the cribriform architecture, where tumor cells form sieve-like structures with luminal spaces.

Immunohistochemistry was performed to further characterize the tumor. The cells were estrogen receptor (ER) positive, progesterone receptor (PR) positive, and HER2/neu negative. This receptor status suggested that the tumor would likely respond to hormonal therapy, providing a glimmer of hope in what was otherwise a grim diagnosis.

Next, we proceeded with staging to assess the extent of disease spread. A contrast-enhanced MRI of the breast was performed, which showed the primary tumor but no evidence of local invasion into the chest wall or skin. A PET-CT scan was conducted to evaluate for distant metastases, which fortunately returned negative. The cancer was classified as Stage IIA (T2N0M0) - a 2.5 cm tumor with no regional lymph node involvement or distant metastasis.

A multidisciplinary team meeting was convened to discuss the optimal treatment approach. The team included surgical oncologists, medical oncologists, radiation oncologists, and a breast cancer nurse specialist. The consensus was to proceed with a modified radical mastectomy followed by adjuvant therapy, given the size of the tumor and the patient's relatively young age.

The patient underwent a modified radical mastectomy, which involves removal of the entire breast tissue along with axillary lymph node dissection. The surgery was uneventful, and the patient was discharged home after a brief hospital stay. Pathological examination of the surgical specimen confirmed the diagnosis of cribriform carcinoma with clear margins. Out of the 12 lymph nodes excised, none showed evidence of metastatic disease, consistent with the earlier staging.

Adjuvant therapy is crucial in reducing the risk of cancer recurrence. Given the hormone receptor-positive status of the tumor, we recommended hormonal therapy with tamoxifen. Tamoxifen acts as an estrogen receptor antagonist in breast tissue, thereby inhibiting the proliferative action of estrogen on malignant cells. The patient was prescribed tamoxifen 20 mg daily for five years, which is the standard duration to achieve maximum benefit.

In addition to hormonal therapy, adjuvant chemotherapy was considered. Although the absence of lymph node involvement suggested a lower risk of recurrence, the relatively young age of the patient and the aggressive nature of cribriform carcinoma warranted a more aggressive approach. A regimen of cyclophosphamide, methotrexate, and fluorouracil (CMF) was chosen, given its efficacy and tolerability profile. The patient underwent six cycles of CMF, administered every three weeks. Throughout the chemotherapy, the patient experienced manageable side effects, including mild nausea, fatigue, and transient neutropenia, which were effectively managed with supportive care.

While the surgical margins were clear, the decision to administer adjuvant radiation therapy was carefully weighed. Radiation therapy can further reduce the risk of local recurrence, especially in patients with large tumors or those with close or positive margins. Given the size of the tumor and the cribriform architecture, which can sometimes exhibit aggressive behavior, adjuvant radiation therapy was recommended. The patient received 50 Gy of radiation to the chest wall over 25 fractions, delivered over five weeks. The treatment was well-tolerated, with only mild erythema and fatigue.

Following the completion of adjuvant therapy, the patient entered the surveillance phase. Regular follow-ups were scheduled every three months for the first two years, then every six months for the next three years, and annually thereafter. Each visit included a thorough physical examination, routine blood tests, and annual mammograms of the contralateral breast.

Despite the comprehensive treatment, cancer recurrence remains a significant concern. Approximately two years after completing adjuvant therapy, the patient reported a new lump in the contralateral breast. A mammogram and ultrasound were promptly performed, revealing a suspicious lesion. A core needle biopsy confirmed the recurrence of cribriform carcinoma. This time, the tumor was 1.8 cm in size and again, hormone receptor-positive.

Given the recurrence, a multidisciplinary team meeting was reconvened. The patient underwent a lumpectomy with sentinel lymph node biopsy, which confirmed the presence of cribriform carcinoma with clear margins and no lymph node involvement. The tumor was staged as Stage IB (T1cN0M0). Given the previous exposure to tamoxifen, the patient was switched to an aromatase inhibitor, letrozole, which is often effective in postmenopausal women or in patients who do not respond to tamoxifen.

Considering the recurrence, additional chemotherapy was discussed. The patient was started on a regimen of doxorubicin and cyclophosphamide followed by paclitaxel. The regimen was chosen based on its efficacy in treating recurrent breast cancer. The patient tolerated the chemotherapy well, with manageable side effects including alopecia, mild neuropathy, and fatigue.

After completing the additional adjuvant therapy, the patient was closely monitored. Follow-up imaging and clinical exams showed no evidence of disease for the next three years. However, during a routine follow-up at the five-year mark, the patient presented with new symptoms, including persistent back pain and unexplained weight loss. A PET-CT scan was performed, revealing multiple osteolytic lesions in the spine and pelvis, consistent with metastatic disease.

A biopsy of one of the bone lesions confirmed metastatic cribriform carcinoma. The prognosis for metastatic breast cancer is generally poor, and treatment focuses on palliative care to manage symptoms and improve quality of life. The patient was started on a regimen of bisphosphonates to strengthen the bones and reduce fracture risk. Additionally, palliative radiation therapy was administered to the spine to alleviate pain.

In the final phase of treatment, the focus shifted to managing symptoms and providing the best possible quality of life. The patient received regular pain management, physical therapy, and psychological support. Despite these efforts, the disease progressed, and the patient eventually succumbed to the complications of metastatic breast cancer.

Cribriform carcinoma, while rare, presents significant challenges in diagnosis and treatment. The patient's journey underscored the importance of a multidisciplinary approach, combining surgery, chemotherapy, radiation, and hormonal therapy to manage the disease.

Despite aggressive treatment, the risk of recurrence and metastasis remains high, highlighting the need for ongoing research and better therapeutic options. The patient's case is a poignant reminder of the relentless nature of cancer and the continuous efforts required in the field of oncology to improve outcomes for future patients.

❧ 17 ❧

HOLMES-ADIE SYNDROME

I remember the patient vividly; they presented to my office with a peculiar set of symptoms that were not immediately recognizable. The initial consultation occurred on an overcast afternoon, with the patient describing a history of blurred vision and an unusual dilation of the right pupil. This was particularly noticeable in bright light, where one would expect the pupil to constrict. Instead, the patient reported that their right pupil remained dilated for an extended period. Additionally, the patient mentioned episodic episodes of an irregular heart rate, which they described as "flutters."

The physical examination confirmed the patient's observations. The right pupil was markedly dilated compared to the left, and the light reflex was sluggish. This asymmetry, known as anisocoria, along with the described visual disturbances and the absence of acute pain or other ocular symptoms, suggested a need for further neurological and ophthalmological investigation.

Holmes-Adie syndrome, or Adie's tonic pupil, was a condition that immediately came to mind. This syndrome is characterized by a tonic pupil that reacts sluggishly to light but accommodates better for near vision and is often accompanied by absent or diminished deep tendon reflexes. However, a definitive diagnosis required more than clinical suspicion.

The next step was to conduct a series of diagnostic tests. A slit-lamp examination revealed segmental palsy of the iris sphincter muscles, a hallmark of the tonic pupil. The patient's pupil constricted sluggishly in response to light but showed a more pronounced response to near vision—classic signs of a tonic pupil. To further confirm the diagnosis, I administered a dilute pilocarpine solution (0.125%) to the affected eye. This test exploits the denervation hypersensitivity of the sphincter muscle in Holmes-Adie syndrome. In a healthy eye, such a low concentration of pilocarpine would have little to no effect. However, in the affected eye of someone with Holmes-Adie syndrome, it causes a noticeable constriction. The patient's right pupil responded significantly to the dilute pilocarpine, supporting the diagnosis.

Given the constellation of symptoms and the confirmatory test results, I diagnosed the patient with Holmes-Adie syndrome. This condition typically affects young adults, with a higher prevalence among females, and often presents unilaterally. The etiology of Holmes-Adie syndrome is thought to involve a viral or bacterial infection that causes inflammation and subsequent damage to the postganglionic fibers of the ciliary ganglion, which innervate the iris sphincter and ciliary muscles. This damage results in the characteristic tonic pupil. The involvement of autonomic nervous system pathways also explains the potential for associated cardiovascular symptoms, such as the irregular heart rate the patient described.

After the diagnosis, we discussed the prognosis and treatment options. Holmes-Adie syndrome is generally benign, and many patients adapt well to their visual disturbances. Treatment is largely symptomatic. For the visual symptoms, corrective lenses can help manage the accommodative issues. Pilocarpine drops can also be used to constrict the pupil temporarily, improving vision in bright light, although long-term use is not generally recommended due to potential side effects and the inconvenience of frequent administration.

For the patient's irregular heart rate, I recommended a cardiology consultation. While the cardiovascular manifestations of Holmes-Adie syndrome are usually benign, it was prudent to rule out other potential causes of the arrhythmias. The cardiologist conducted an electrocardiogram (ECG) and a Holter monitor study to evaluate the patient's heart rhythm over a 24-hour period. The results showed sporadic episodes of premature ventricular contractions (PVCs), which were deemed benign and not requiring specific treatment beyond monitoring.

In terms of managing the syndrome itself, I emphasized the importance of regular follow-ups to monitor any progression of symptoms or the emergence of new signs. Additionally, I informed the patient about the possibility of the syndrome affecting the other eye, although this occurs in a minority of cases.

As time went on, the patient adjusted to their condition with a combination of adaptive strategies and minor medical interventions. They used tinted lenses to reduce the impact of light sensitivity, and on particularly troublesome days, they applied pilocarpine drops under guidance. The patient's heart irregularities remained benign, and the cardiologist's follow-ups confirmed that no further intervention was necessary.

Over the course of a year, the patient adapted well to the visual disturbances and their episodic heart irregularities. The tonic pupil's response became a part of their daily life, and they reported fewer issues as they learned to manage the symptoms effectively. The follow-up consultations were routine, with no significant changes in the patient's condition.

Then, approximately eighteen months after the

initial diagnosis, the patient presented with new symptoms. They reported numbness and tingling in the extremities, as well as a noticeable weakness in the legs. Given these new neurological symptoms, I ordered a series of tests to rule out other potential causes and to understand if there was any link to the existing Holmes-Adie diagnosis.

A comprehensive neurological examination was performed, including electromyography (EMG) and nerve conduction studies. These tests revealed peripheral neuropathy, characterized by a decrease in nerve conduction velocity and abnormal EMG results. This suggested an additional layer of complexity in the patient's condition, potentially indicating an overlap with another neurological disorder.

Given the new symptoms and findings, I consulted with a neurologist to explore potential connections and to rule out other conditions such as autoimmune disorders, which can sometimes present with overlapping symptoms. The neurologist recommended further testing, including blood tests for autoimmune markers and a lumbar puncture to analyze cerebrospinal fluid.

The test results came back negative for any markers of autoimmune disease, and the cerebrospinal fluid analysis showed no signs of infection or inflammation. The peripheral neuropathy was thus considered idiopathic, potentially a secondary manifestation of the patient's Holmes-Adie syndrome or another benign process.

The patient's treatment plan was adjusted to address these new symptoms. Physical therapy was recommended to help manage the muscle weakness and improve mobility. Additionally, medications such as gabapentin were prescribed to help alleviate the neuropathic pain and discomfort.

Despite these additional challenges, the patient's overall health remained stable. They continued with regular follow-ups, and their quality of life was carefully monitored and managed. The patient's vision remained stable, and their heart irregularities did not worsen. The peripheral neuropathy symptoms were managed effectively with the prescribed treatments.

In the ensuing years, the patient remained under periodic observation. Their condition remained stable, with no significant progression of symptoms. The visual disturbances caused by the tonic pupil were well managed, and the heart irregularities remained benign. The peripheral neuropathy, while a source of discomfort, was effectively managed with medication and physical therapy.

In summary, the patient's journey with Holmes-Adie syndrome was marked by an initial period of adjustment followed by the emergence of additional neurological symptoms. Through a combination of diagnostic vigilance, symptomatic treatment, and regular follow-ups, the patient managed to lead a stable life despite the chronic nature of their condition. This case underscored the importance of a comprehensive approach to diagnosis and treatment, as well as the need for ongoing management in chronic neurological conditions.

✵ 18 ✵

KUFS DISEASE

The patient came to my office complaining of increasing difficulty with coordination and muscle weakness. Initially, I considered more common neurodegenerative disorders such as Parkinson's disease or multiple sclerosis. However, upon conducting a thorough examination and noting the patient's symptoms, I suspected a more rare condition. The patient exhibited symptoms such as seizures, vision problems, and behavioral changes that did not fit neatly into the more common diagnoses.

Given the constellation of symptoms, I ordered a series of tests, starting with a full neurological examination and MRI scan of the brain. The MRI revealed atrophy in the brain's cerebellum and changes in the basal ganglia, which were unusual and pointed toward a metabolic or storage disorder. Additionally, I noticed pigmentary retinopathy upon a detailed eye examination, which further indicated a possible diagnosis of neuronal ceroid lipofuscinosis (NCL), a group of disorders characterized by the accumulation of lipofuscin in the body's tissues.

To confirm my suspicions, I recommended genetic testing and an enzyme assay. The genetic test identified mutations in the CLN6 gene, which are known to cause Kufs disease, a form of adult-onset NCL. The enzyme assay showed reduced activity of specific enzymes typically associated with lysosomal storage disorders, which further supported the diagnosis of Kufs disease.

Kufs disease, or adult-onset neuronal ceroid lipofuscinosis, is a rare, inherited disorder that affects the nervous system. It is part of a group of disorders known as neuronal ceroid lipofuscinoses, characterized by the accumulation of lipofuscin—a fatty, pigmented substance —in the body's tissues. These accumulations primarily affect the brain, leading to a variety of neurological symptoms.

After confirming the diagnosis, I discussed the prognosis and treatment options with the patient and their family. Unfortunately, there is no cure for Kufs disease, and treatment is primarily supportive and aimed at managing symptoms. This includes medications to control seizures, physical therapy to help with muscle coordination and strength, and psychiatric support to address behavioral changes and cognitive decline.

The patient was started on a regimen of antiepileptic drugs (AEDs) to control the seizures. These medications included levetiracetam and lamotrigine, chosen for their effectiveness and relatively favorable side effect profile. Monitoring the patient closely, we adjusted the dosages to achieve optimal seizure control while minimizing adverse effects.

In addition to AEDs, the patient was prescribed medications to address muscle rigidity and spasticity. Baclofen and tizanidine were utilized to help manage these symptoms. Regular physical therapy sessions were arranged to help maintain as much muscle function and coordination as possible. The physical therapist worked on exercises to improve balance, strength, and coordination, which could help slow the progression of motor symptoms.

The patient's vision problems were managed with the help of an ophthalmologist. Regular eye examinations were scheduled, and visual aids were provided to help the patient maintain independence in daily activities. The pigmentary retinopathy caused by the accumulation of lipofuscin in the retinal cells was monitored, although no specific treatment could reverse the damage.

Cognitive and behavioral changes were addressed through psychiatric support and medication. The patient exhibited symptoms of depression and anxiety, common in individuals with neurodegenerative diseases. Antidepressants such as sertraline were prescribed to help manage these symptoms. Counseling and support groups were also recommended to provide emotional support for both the patient and their family.

As the disease progressed, the patient's symptoms became more pronounced. The seizures, despite medication, became harder to control and more frequent. The patient's cognitive functions declined, leading to significant memory loss and difficulty performing daily tasks. The family was provided with resources and support for caregiving, including training on how to assist with activities of daily living and manage behavioral issues.

Despite the best efforts, the patient's condition continued to deteriorate. The accumulation of lipofuscin in the brain cells led to increasing neurological impairment. The patient experienced more frequent and severe seizures, often requiring hospitalization. Muscle weakness and coordination problems worsened, confining the patient to a wheelchair.

Throughout the course of the disease, I closely monitored the patient's condition and made adjustments to the treatment plan as needed. We tried various combinations of medications to control seizures and manage other symptoms, but the progressive nature of Kufs disease meant that our efforts could only slow, not halt, the decline.

The patient's family was incredibly supportive, ensuring that the patient received the best care possible at home. We arranged for home healthcare services to assist with daily care and provide respite for the family. Despite these measures, the patient's quality of life continued to decline.

In the final stages of the disease, the patient became bedridden. Seizures were frequent and severe, and the patient's cognitive functions were significantly impaired. The patient required round-the-clock care and assistance with all activities of daily living. Pain management became a focus of care, with medications adjusted to ensure the patient was as comfortable as possible.

The patient succumbed to the disease after several years of progressive decline. Kufs disease, like other forms of neuronal ceroid lipofuscinosis, is relentlessly progressive and ultimately fatal. The accumulation of lipofuscin in the brain and other tissues leads to a cascade of neurological dysfunctions that cannot be reversed.

Reflecting on the patient's case, I was reminded of the challenges we face in treating rare neurodegenerative diseases. The lack of a cure and the limited treatment options highlight the need for continued research into these devastating conditions. The patient's journey, though marked by suffering, also demonstrated the resilience of the human spirit and the importance of compassionate care in the face of incurable illness.

Kufs disease remains a rare and poorly understood condition, with much of the pathophysiology still unknown. It is believed to result from mutations in genes involved in lysosomal function, leading to the accumulation of lipofuscin. This accumulation disrupts normal cellular function, particularly in neurons, leading to the progressive neurological symptoms observed in patients.

Genetic research continues to uncover new information about the various forms of neuronal ceroid lipofuscinosis, including Kufs disease. Advances in gene therapy and molecular medicine hold promise for future treatments, but as of now, these remain in the experimental stages.

In the clinical setting, managing a patient with Kufs disease involves a multidisciplinary approach. Neurologists, ophthalmologists, psychiatrists, and physical therapists all play crucial roles in providing comprehensive care. Regular follow-up and adjustments to the treatment plan are necessary to address the evolving symptoms and complications.

The patient's case underscored the importance of early and accurate diagnosis. Genetic testing and enzyme assays were critical in identifying Kufs disease and distinguishing it from other neurodegenerative disorders. Early diagnosis allows for better planning and management of the disease, although the ultimate prognosis remains poor.

Throughout the patient's illness, support for the family was also a key aspect of care. Caregiving for a patient with a progressive neurodegenerative disease is incredibly demanding, both physically and emotionally. Providing resources, education, and emotional support for caregivers is essential to ensure they can continue to care for their loved ones and maintain their well-being.

In conclusion, the patient's journey through Kufs disease was marked by progressive neurological decline and increasing dependence on care. Despite the lack of curative treatments, the multidisciplinary care approach aimed to manage symptoms and maintain the best possible quality of life. The case highlighted the need for continued research into rare neurodegenerative diseases and the importance of compassionate, comprehensive care for patients and their families. The patient's story is a testament to the resilience of those affected by such diseases and the ongoing efforts of the medical community to provide support and care in the face of significant challenges.

19

POLYGLUCOSAN BODY DISEASE

P olyglucosan body disease (PBD) is a rare, inherited disorder characterized by the accumulation of abnormal glycogen within cells. This glycogen, known as polyglucosan, disrupts normal cellular function, leading to a variety of symptoms, often affecting the nervous system. As a neurologist, I encountered a particularly challenging case of PBD, which provided significant insights into the disease's diagnosis, treatment, and progression.

The patient, a 56-year-old male, presented with progressive weakness, difficulty walking, and cognitive decline over the past few years. His medical history was unremarkable, and there was no known family history of similar conditions. Upon initial examination, the patient exhibited significant motor dysfunction, including spasticity and weakness in the lower limbs, as well as mild cognitive impairment. Reflexes were brisk, and Babinski sign was positive. These findings suggested a neurological disorder affecting both the central and peripheral nervous systems.

Given the progressive nature of the symptoms, we initiated a comprehensive diagnostic workup. Initial blood tests, including complete blood count, liver function tests, and thyroid function tests, were within normal limits. Vitamin B12 and folate levels were also normal, ruling out common metabolic causes of neurological decline. MRI of the brain and spinal cord was performed, revealing diffuse white matter hyperintensities, particularly in the periventricular and subcortical regions. These findings were non-specific but suggested a neurodegenerative process.

To further narrow down the differential diagnosis, we performed cerebrospinal fluid (CSF) analysis through a lumbar puncture. The CSF analysis showed mildly elevated protein levels but no oligoclonal bands, ruling out multiple sclerosis. Nerve conduction studies and electromyography (EMG) were performed to assess peripheral nerve function. These tests revealed reduced nerve conduction velocities and evidence of chronic denervation, indicating a peripheral neuropathy component.

Given the combination of central and peripheral nervous system involvement, we considered several possible diagnoses, including leukodystrophies, mitochondrial disorders, and glycogen storage diseases. To explore these possibilities, we ordered a series of genetic tests. Whole exome sequencing was conducted, and the results revealed a mutation in the GBE1 gene, confirming the diagnosis of adult polyglucosan body disease (APBD). This mutation leads to a deficiency in the enzyme glycogen branching enzyme, which is crucial for proper glycogen synthesis.

With the diagnosis confirmed, we turned our attention to management and treatment. Unfortunately, there is no cure for APBD, and treatment is primarily supportive and aimed at managing symptoms. We assembled a multidisciplinary team, including neurologists, physiotherapists, occupational therapists, and a genetic counselor, to provide comprehensive care.

For the motor symptoms, we initiated a regimen of physical therapy to maintain muscle strength and improve mobility. The patient participated in regular exercises focused on strengthening the lower limbs and improving balance. Additionally, we prescribed baclofen to manage spasticity and reduce muscle stiffness. The patient was also provided with assistive devices, such as a walker, to aid in mobility and prevent falls.

Cognitive decline was addressed through cognitive rehabilitation therapy. This included memory exercises, problem-solving tasks, and strategies to improve daily functioning. We also monitored the patient for signs of depression and anxiety, which are common in individuals with chronic neurodegenerative diseases. Antidepressant medication was prescribed as needed.

Given the patient's progressive peripheral neuropathy, we recommended regular follow-up with a neurologist specializing in neuromuscular disorders. Pain management was an important aspect of care, as neuropathic pain can be debilitating. We prescribed gabapentin, which provided some relief from the burning and tingling sensations in the extremities.

In addition to symptomatic treatment, we explored experimental therapies. Research on APBD is ongoing, and several potential treatments are under investigation. One such treatment involves enzyme replacement therapy (ERT) aimed at supplementing the deficient glycogen branching enzyme. Although ERT is still in the experimental stage, we discussed the possibility of enrolling the patient in a clinical trial. After careful consideration, the patient agreed to participate in a trial, which provided hope for a potential breakthrough in treatment.

As part of the clinical trial, the patient received intravenous infusions of the recombinant glycogen branching enzyme every two weeks. Regular assessments were conducted to monitor the effectiveness of the treatment and any adverse effects. Over the course of several months, we observed some stabilization of the patient's motor symptoms. While the progression of weakness and spasticity slowed, there was no significant improvement in cognitive function.

The clinical trial also included regular imaging studies, such as MRI and PET scans, to assess changes in brain structure and function. These scans revealed a slight reduction in the extent of white matter abnormalities, suggesting a potential benefit of the enzyme replacement therapy. However, the long-term efficacy and safety of this treatment remained uncertain.

In addition to medical management, we emphasized the importance of genetic counseling for the patient and his family. APBD is an autosomal recessive disorder, meaning both parents must carry a copy of the mutated gene for a child to be affected. Genetic counseling provided information about the risk of passing the condition to future generations and offered options for family planning, including preimplantation genetic diagnosis (PGD) for those considering having children.

As the disease progressed, the patient's mobility continued to decline, necessitating the use of a wheelchair. Despite these challenges, the patient remained determined to maintain his independence and quality of life. We worked closely with occupational therapists to adapt the patient's home environment, ensuring it was wheelchair accessible and equipped with assistive devices to facilitate daily activities.

Over the following year, the patient's condition remained relatively stable. However, as is often the case with neurodegenerative diseases, complications arose. The patient developed recurrent urinary tract infections due to neurogenic bladder dysfunction. This required intermittent catheterization and prophylactic antibiotics to prevent further infections.

The patient's nutritional status also became a concern. Progressive dysphagia, or difficulty swallowing, led to weight loss and malnutrition. We consulted with a dietitian to develop a high-calorie, easy-to-swallow diet plan. In severe cases, a feeding tube may be necessary, but we aimed to delay this intervention as long as possible to preserve the patient's quality of life.

Unfortunately, despite our best efforts, the patient's condition continued to deteriorate. Respiratory complications emerged due to weakening of the respiratory muscles. The patient experienced frequent respiratory infections and required non-invasive ventilation support at night to assist with breathing. These complications marked a significant decline in the patient's overall health.

Approximately three years after the initial diagnosis, the patient's condition reached a critical point. The progression of the disease led to severe respiratory failure, and the patient was admitted to the intensive care unit (ICU). Despite aggressive medical intervention, including mechanical ventilation, the patient's condition continued to worsen. After extensive discussions with the family about the patient's wishes and quality of life considerations, a decision was made to withdraw life-sustaining treatment.

The patient passed away peacefully, surrounded by family. This case of APBD highlighted the challenges of managing a rare and progressive neurodegenerative disease. While there were moments of hope with experimental therapies and supportive care, the inexorable progression of the disease ultimately led to a terminal outcome.

In reflecting on this case, several key points emerge. Early diagnosis of APBD is crucial, as it allows for timely intervention and management of symptoms. Genetic testing plays a vital role in identifying the underlying cause and guiding treatment decisions. Multidisciplinary care is essential to address the complex needs of patients with APBD, involving neurologists, physiotherapists, occupational therapists, dietitians, and genetic counselors.

Research into novel therapies, such as enzyme replacement therapy, offers hope for the future. Although the clinical trial in this case did not lead to a cure, it provided valuable insights into the potential benefits and limitations of such treatments. Continued research and participation in clinical trials are essential to advance our understanding of APBD and develop effective treatments.

Lastly, the importance of palliative care and end-of-life planning cannot be overstated. As APBD progresses, addressing the patient's comfort and quality of life becomes paramount. Engaging in open and compassionate discussions with patients and their families about their wishes and goals of care is essential in providing holistic and patient-centered care.

20

WISSLER-FANCONI SYNDROME

Wissler-Fanconi syndrome, an extremely rare disorder, presented itself to me in the form of a young patient whose case would become etched in my memory due to its complexity and the profound challenges it posed. The syndrome, characterized by symptoms reminiscent of both rheumatoid arthritis and systemic lupus erythematosus (SLE), required careful diagnostic acumen and a robust treatment plan to manage.

The patient first presented with a high fever, which had been persistent for over two weeks. This was accompanied by joint pain, predominantly in the knees and wrists, and a notable rash that had spread across the chest and upper arms. Initially, these symptoms suggested a viral infection or a form of juvenile idiopathic arthritis. However, the persistence and severity of the symptoms prompted further investigation.

A comprehensive physical examination revealed several key findings. The patient exhibited marked swelling and tenderness in multiple joints, notably the knees, wrists, and fingers. The rash, erythematous and slightly raised, did not blanch under pressure, suggesting an inflammatory etiology. Additionally, there was a noticeable paleness to the skin, indicating possible anemia.

Given the constellation of symptoms, we ordered a battery of tests. Initial blood work showed elevated inflammatory markers, including C-reactive protein (CRP) and erythrocyte sedimentation rate (ESR). A complete blood count (CBC) revealed significant leukocytosis and anemia. Renal function tests showed elevated creatinine and blood urea nitrogen (BUN) levels, indicating potential kidney involvement. Urinalysis revealed proteinuria and hematuria, further supporting renal involvement.

Given the overlapping features of systemic autoimmune disorders, we proceeded with serological testing. The antinuclear antibody (ANA) test returned positive with a high titer, and further testing showed the presence of anti-double-stranded DNA (anti-dsDNA) antibodies. Rheumatoid factor (RF) was negative, but anti-cyclic citrullinated peptide (anti-CCP) antibodies were positive. These results, combined with the clinical presentation, strongly suggested a diagnosis of Wissler-Fanconi syndrome, a rare overlap syndrome with features of both rheumatoid arthritis and lupus.

The treatment approach for Wissler-Fanconi syndrome required a multi-faceted strategy to manage the autoimmune response and address the systemic involvement, particularly the renal complications. Given the severity of the symptoms and the risk of progression, we opted for an aggressive initial treatment plan.

1. Immunosuppressive Therapy:

To control the autoimmune activity, we initiated high-dose corticosteroids. Prednisone was administered at a dose of 1 mg/kg/day, which was intended to rapidly reduce inflammation and prevent further joint and organ damage. The patient responded moderately to the corticosteroids, with a reduction in fever and joint pain, but renal function continued to decline.

Given the partial response, we introduced additional immunosuppressive agents. Methotrexate, a disease-modifying antirheumatic drug (DMARD), was started at 15 mg/week, gradually increasing to 20 mg/week based on tolerance. Methotrexate helps to suppress the overactive immune response and slow disease progression. Concurrently, we added mycophenolate mofetil (MMF) at a dose of 1 g twice daily, which has shown efficacy in lupus nephritis and other autoimmune disorders involving the kidneys.

2. Renal Protection and Management:

With the patient's renal function deteriorating, we consulted with a nephrologist. The patient was started on angiotensin-converting enzyme (ACE) inhibitors, specifically enalapril at 10 mg/day, to help reduce proteinuria and protect renal function. Additionally, we closely monitored renal function through regular blood tests and urine analysis.

The nephrologist recommended the addition of plasmapheresis, a procedure to remove antibodies from the blood, in hopes of reducing the autoimmune attack on the kidneys. The patient underwent plasmapheresis sessions every other day for two weeks. This intervention showed some improvement in renal parameters, with a slight reduction in creatinine levels and proteinuria.

3. Supportive Care:

Given the significant anemia, we initiated treatment with erythropoiesis-stimulating agents (ESAs) to stimulate red blood cell production. The patient received darbepoetin alfa at a dose of 0.45 mcg/kg every two weeks. Additionally, iron supplementation was provided intravenously to address iron deficiency, which was confirmed by serum ferritin and transferrin saturation tests.

Pain management was another crucial aspect of care. Nonsteroidal anti-inflammatory drugs (NSAIDs) were initially used, but given the renal involvement, we switched to acetaminophen for pain relief. Opioid analgesics were avoided due to their potential side effects and the risk of dependency.

4. Monitoring and Adjustments:

Over the course of the treatment, we closely monitored the patient's response through regular blood tests, urine analysis, and imaging studies. Adjustments were made based on the clinical response and side effects. For instance, methotrexate dosage was adjusted to manage gastrointestinal side effects, and additional folic acid supplementation was provided to mitigate the risk of methotrexate-induced folate deficiency.

Despite the aggressive treatment, the patient's response was mixed. The fever and joint pain showed significant improvement, and the rash resolved completely. However, renal function remained a major concern. The initial improvement in renal parameters following plasmapheresis plateaued, and subsequent tests showed a gradual decline in renal function.

After three months of treatment, the patient developed worsening renal failure, evidenced by rising creatinine and BUN levels, and an increase in proteinuria. The nephrologist recommended a kidney biopsy to assess the extent of damage and guide further treatment. The biopsy revealed advanced glomerulonephritis with extensive scarring, indicative of chronic damage that was unlikely to be reversible.

Given the prognosis, we discussed the next steps with the patient and their family. The nephrologist advised considering dialysis to manage the renal failure and maintain quality of life. After thorough discussions and considering the patient's wishes, we initiated hemodialysis. The patient received dialysis three times a week, which helped to manage the symptoms of renal failure, including fluid overload and electrolyte imbalances.

Over the next several months, the patient's condition remained stable but fragile. The autoimmune activity was well-controlled with the ongoing use of methotrexate and mycophenolate mofetil, and corticosteroids were gradually tapered to a maintenance dose. However, the chronic renal failure persisted, requiring continuous dialysis.

Unfortunately, the patient developed complications associated with long-term dialysis, including access site infections and cardiovascular issues. Despite aggressive management, these complications took a toll on the patient's overall health.

After 18 months of treatment, the patient's condition deteriorated further. They developed severe sepsis due to an infected dialysis catheter, which led to multi-organ failure. Despite intensive care and aggressive antibiotic therapy, the patient succumbed to septic shock.

The case of Wissler-Fanconi syndrome in this patient highlighted the severe and complex nature of this rare autoimmune disorder. Despite an aggressive and multi-faceted treatment approach, the patient's renal involvement proved to be the most challenging aspect to manage. The progression to chronic renal failure and the subsequent complications associated with long-term dialysis ultimately led to a fatal outcome.

This case underscored the importance of early diagnosis and aggressive management in autoimmune disorders with multi-organ involvement. It also highlighted the need for ongoing research to better understand and develop targeted therapies for rare conditions like Wissler-Fanconi syndrome. The lessons learned from this case will inform future management strategies and underscore the need for a multidisciplinary approach in managing complex autoimmune diseases.

❧ 21 ❧

ACROMEGALY

When the patient first walked into my office, it was impossible to ignore the prominent features that marked their condition. Enlarged hands, a protruding jaw, and coarse facial features were all hallmarks of Acromegaly. I immediately suspected the diagnosis but needed a thorough evaluation to confirm it.

The patient described a range of symptoms that had been progressively worsening over the past few years. They reported experiencing frequent headaches, joint pain, and excessive sweating. Additionally, they mentioned that their shoe and ring sizes had increased, which is a common indication of the underlying disorder. The patient's history of changes in physical appearance and the symptoms they described were strongly suggestive of Acromegaly, a disorder caused by excessive secretion of growth hormone (GH), typically due to a pituitary adenoma.

To confirm the diagnosis, I ordered a series of tests. The first step was to measure the levels of insulin-like growth factor 1 (IGF-1) in the patient's blood. IGF-1 levels are typically elevated in patients with Acromegaly and are a reliable indicator of GH activity. The results came back significantly above the normal range, corroborating my initial suspicion.

Next, I performed an oral glucose tolerance test (OGTT). In a healthy individual, glucose ingestion suppresses GH secretion. However, in patients with Acromegaly, this suppression does not occur, and GH levels remain elevated. As expected, the patient's GH levels did not decrease after glucose ingestion, further confirming the diagnosis.

The final step in the diagnostic process was imaging. Magnetic resonance imaging (MRI) of the pituitary gland was performed to visualize the presence of a pituitary adenoma. The MRI revealed a 1.5 cm tumor in the anterior pituitary, consistent with a growth hormone-secreting adenoma. With these findings, the diagnosis of Acromegaly was definitive.

Having confirmed the diagnosis, the next step was to discuss treatment options with the patient. The primary goal in treating Acromegaly is to normalize GH and IGF-1 levels, reduce tumor size, alleviate symptoms, and prevent complications. The treatment plan would involve a combination of surgery, medication, and potentially radiation therapy.

The first-line treatment for most patients with Acromegaly is transsphenoidal surgery to remove the pituitary adenoma. This minimally invasive procedure involves accessing the pituitary gland through the nasal passages. The patient was referred to a skilled neurosurgeon who had extensive experience with this type of surgery.

The surgery was scheduled, and preoperative assessments were conducted to ensure the patient was fit for the procedure. The surgical team carefully explained the risks and benefits, emphasizing that while surgery had a high success rate, there was no guarantee that all tumor cells would be removed or that GH levels would normalize immediately.

On the day of the surgery, the patient was prepped, and the neurosurgeon performed the transsphenoidal resection of the pituitary adenoma. The operation was successful, with the surgeon reporting that they were able to remove the tumor entirely. Postoperative monitoring was crucial to assess the immediate outcomes of the surgery.

In the days following the surgery, the patient's GH and IGF-1 levels were closely monitored. Initial postoperative tests showed a significant reduction in GH levels, but they were still above the normal range. This indicated that while the tumor had been successfully removed, the patient would likely require adjunctive therapy to achieve biochemical remission.

The next step in the treatment plan was the introduction of medication. The patient was started on a somatostatin analog, specifically octreotide, which helps to suppress GH secretion. Octreotide injections were administered, and the patient's hormone levels were monitored regularly. Over the next few months, the patient's IGF-1 levels gradually approached the normal range, and their symptoms began to improve.

Despite the improvements, the patient's GH levels remained slightly elevated. To address this, the treatment regimen was adjusted to include pegvisomant, a GH receptor antagonist. Pegvisomant works by blocking the effects of GH at the receptor level, thereby reducing IGF-1 production. This combination therapy proved effective, and subsequent tests showed that both GH and IGF-1 levels were within the normal range.

However, achieving biochemical remission did not immediately resolve all of the patient's symptoms. The patient continued to experience joint pain and required additional management for osteoarthritis, a common complication of Acromegaly. Physical therapy was introduced to help alleviate the pain and improve joint function. Additionally, the patient was monitored for other potential complications, such as cardiovascular issues and diabetes, which are more prevalent in individuals with Acromegaly.

Despite the successful biochemical management of the condition, the patient also faced psychological challenges. The changes in their physical appearance had taken a toll on their mental health, leading to issues with self-esteem and depression. A referral to a mental health professional was made, and the patient received counseling and support to help cope with these challenges.

Over the next year, the patient showed remarkable progress. Regular follow-up appointments were scheduled to monitor hormone levels and overall health. MRI scans were performed periodically to ensure there was no recurrence of the pituitary adenoma. The combination of surgery, medication, and supportive therapies had brought the patient's Acromegaly under control.

In the long term, the patient remained stable with normalized GH and IGF-1 levels. The physical symptoms, such as joint pain, persisted but were managed effectively with ongoing physical therapy and pain management strategies. The patient's cardiovascular health was closely monitored, and lifestyle modifications were recommended to mitigate any risks.

The case of this patient highlights the complexities and challenges of managing Acromegaly. While the primary goal of treatment was achieved—normalizing hormone levels and removing the adenoma—the journey to manage and support the patient's overall well-being was multifaceted. This included addressing the physical complications of the disease, providing psychological support, and ensuring continuous monitoring to prevent recurrence or new complications.

In summary, the patient was diagnosed with Acromegaly through a combination of clinical evaluation, biochemical testing, and imaging studies. Treatment involved successful transsphenoidal surgery to remove the pituitary adenoma, followed by medication to normalize hormone levels. The patient experienced significant improvements but required ongoing management for persistent symptoms and complications. Ultimately, the multidisciplinary approach led to a successful outcome, with the patient achieving biochemical remission and an improved quality of life.

The patient first came to my attention when they were referred to our specialized genetic disorders clinic by a pediatrician concerned about their abnormal growth patterns and a suite of other troubling symptoms. The patient was a 5-year-old child who had been experiencing progressive symptoms that included short stature, coarse facial features, and joint stiffness. The pediatrician had suspected a mucopolysaccharidosis (MPS) disorder, given the constellation of symptoms, and had requested further genetic and enzymatic analysis.

Upon initial examination, the patient presented with several classic phenotypic characteristics of MPS disorders. The patient was below the 5th percentile for height and had notable dysmorphic facial features, including a prominent forehead, depressed nasal bridge, and macroglossia. Additionally, the patient exhibited limited range of motion in their shoulders and hips, and the parents reported a history of recurrent ear infections and chronic nasal congestion.

Given the clinical presentation, our next step was to confirm the diagnosis through biochemical assays and genetic testing. We obtained blood samples to measure the activity of the enzyme arylsulfatase B (ARSB), which is deficient in Maroteaux-Lamy syndrome (MPS VI). We also performed a urine test to check for elevated levels of dermatan sulfate, a glycosaminoglycan that accumulates in patients with MPS VI due to the deficiency of ARSB.

The enzymatic assay results were unequivocal. The patient's ARSB activity was significantly reduced, measuring less than 10% of the normal reference range. The urine glycosaminoglycan analysis showed markedly elevated dermatan sulfate levels, further supporting our clinical suspicion. To definitively confirm the diagnosis, we proceeded with genetic testing, which identified two pathogenic variants in the ARSB gene, consistent with a diagnosis of Maroteaux-Lamy syndrome.

With the diagnosis confirmed, we discussed the treatment options with the patient's parents. Maroteaux-Lamy syndrome is a progressive disorder that, if left untreated, leads to severe morbidity and early mortality. The mainstay of treatment for MPS VI is enzyme replacement therapy (ERT), which involves regular infusions of recombinant human arylsulfatase B (rhARSB). The goal of ERT is to replace the deficient enzyme and reduce the accumulation of dermatan sulfate in tissues, thereby slowing the progression of the disease and alleviating symptoms.

We initiated the patient on weekly infusions of rhARSB at a dose of 1 mg/kg. The infusions were administered in our clinic under close supervision to monitor for potential infusion-related reactions, which can include fever, chills, and allergic responses. To mitigate the risk of these reactions, we premedicated the patient with antihistamines and acetaminophen prior to each infusion.

Over the first few months of treatment, we closely monitored the patient's clinical status and biochemical markers. The patient tolerated the infusions well, with no significant adverse reactions. Clinically, we observed improvements in the patient's energy levels and a reduction in the frequency of upper respiratory infections. The parents reported that the patient was more active and could participate in physical activities with less discomfort.

Biochemical monitoring showed a gradual decline in urinary dermatan sulfate levels, indicating that the ERT was effectively reducing the storage material in the patient's tissues. We also performed periodic imaging studies, including echocardiograms and MRI scans, to assess the impact of treatment on the patient's organs. The echocardiograms showed stabilization of cardiac valve thickening, a common complication in MPS VI, and the MRI scans revealed no progression of spinal cord compression, another serious concern in this disorder.

As the patient continued ERT, we also addressed other supportive care needs. We referred the patient to an orthopedic specialist for management of joint stiffness and to an otolaryngologist for evaluation of chronic ear infections and potential hearing loss. The orthopedic specialist recommended physical therapy to improve joint mobility and prevent contractures, while the otolaryngologist performed tympanostomy tube placement to alleviate chronic otitis media.

Throughout the course of treatment, we emphasized the importance of regular follow-up visits to monitor the patient's response to therapy and to address any emerging complications. Maroteaux-Lamy syndrome requires a multidisciplinary approach, and we coordinated care with various specialists to provide comprehensive management.

Despite the improvements with ERT, it is important to recognize that enzyme replacement therapy does not cross the blood-brain barrier, and thus, it does not address the central nervous system manifestations of MPS VI. While our patient did not exhibit significant neurological symptoms at the time of diagnosis, we remained vigilant for any signs of cognitive decline or spinal cord involvement, which could necessitate additional interventions such as hematopoietic stem cell transplantation (HSCT).

Over the next few years, the patient remained on ERT with continued clinical benefits. Growth velocity improved, although the patient remained short-statured compared to age-matched peers. Joint mobility was maintained, and the frequency of respiratory infections remained low. Cardiac function was stable, with no further progression of valve thickening.

However, as the patient approached adolescence, we encountered new challenges. The patient began to experience increasing pain and stiffness in the joints, particularly the hips and knees. Radiographic imaging revealed the development of hip dysplasia and femoral head avascular necrosis, complications that are not uncommon in MPS VI due to abnormal bone and cartilage development. The orthopedic team recommended surgical intervention to address these issues, and the patient underwent a series of orthopedic surgeries to improve joint function and alleviate pain.

Postoperative recovery was challenging, requiring intensive physical therapy and pain management. We worked closely with the orthopedic and physical therapy teams to optimize the patient's rehabilitation and ensure the best possible functional outcomes. Despite these efforts, the patient's mobility remained limited, and they required assistive devices for ambulation.

Throughout this period, we continued ERT and monitored the patient's overall health. Routine assessments included echocardiograms, pulmonary function tests, and neuroimaging studies to detect any potential complications. Fortunately, there were no significant cardiac or pulmonary issues, and the patient's cognitive function remained intact.

As the patient transitioned into adulthood, we focused on ensuring a smooth transfer of care to adult services. We facilitated referrals to adult geneticists, cardiologists, and orthopedists to provide ongoing management of MPS VI. We also discussed reproductive counseling, as individuals with MPS VI can have children, and it is important for them to understand the genetic implications and potential risks to offspring.

Despite the many challenges and interventions, the patient's quality of life was relatively good. The patient completed high school with accommodations for physical limitations and pursued higher education with a focus on a career that would be compatible with their abilities. The patient's determination and resilience were truly remarkable, and they became an advocate for others with rare genetic disorders.

As the patient continued with their enzyme replacement therapy, we faced ongoing issues that required vigilance and quick adaptation. One significant concern that emerged was the potential development of spinal cord compression due to the accumulation of glycosaminoglycans around the spinal cord. This complication can result in severe neurological deficits if not promptly identified and managed.

Regular MRI scans of the spine were scheduled to monitor for any signs of compression. At one point, imaging revealed early indications of cervical spinal cord compression. While the patient was not yet symptomatic, this finding necessitated a proactive approach. We referred the patient to a neurosurgeon with experience in managing mucopolysaccharidosis-related spinal issues. The neurosurgeon recommended surgical decompression to prevent future neurological complications.

The patient underwent a cervical laminectomy, a procedure aimed at relieving pressure on the spinal cord. The surgery was successful, and the patient's postoperative recovery was closely monitored. Physical therapy played a crucial role in the patient's rehabilitation, focusing on maintaining and improving strength and mobility.

Another area of concern was the development of corneal clouding, a common ocular manifestation in Maroteaux-Lamy syndrome. This condition results from the accumulation of glycosaminoglycans in the cornea, leading to decreased visual acuity. Regular ophthalmologic evaluations were conducted to assess the severity of corneal clouding and determine the need for intervention.

As the patient's corneal clouding progressed, it became evident that visual impairment was impacting their quality of life. The ophthalmologist recommended a corneal transplant to restore vision. The patient underwent the transplant procedure, which significantly improved visual acuity. Postoperative care included immunosuppressive therapy to prevent graft rejection, and the patient's vision remained stable following the surgery.

Throughout the patient's adolescence and early adulthood, maintaining social and emotional well-being was as important as managing physical health. Living with a chronic genetic disorder posed numerous challenges, including coping with physical limitations and the psychological impact of the disease. We referred the patient to a psychologist specializing in chronic illness to provide support and counseling.

The psychologist worked with the patient on developing coping strategies and addressing the emotional aspects of living with Maroteaux-Lamy syndrome. Support groups and connecting with other individuals facing similar challenges also played a crucial role in the patient's emotional well-being.

In addition to medical and psychological support,

ensuring access to educational accommodations was vital for the patient's academic success. We worked with the patient's school to implement individualized education plans (IEPs) that addressed physical and learning needs. This included accommodations such as extended time for exams, access to assistive technology, and modifications to the physical environment to ensure accessibility.

As the patient transitioned to higher education, similar accommodations were arranged with the university. The patient pursued a degree in a field that aligned with their interests and abilities, demonstrating remarkable determination and resilience. Their academic achievements and advocacy efforts inspired others in the rare disease community.

One of the critical aspects of managing Maroteaux-Lamy syndrome is ensuring continuity of care as the patient transitions from pediatric to adult healthcare services. This transition can be challenging, as adult healthcare providers may have limited experience with rare genetic disorders. To facilitate a smooth transition, we developed a comprehensive transition plan that included detailed medical records, a summary of ongoing treatment and management strategies, and referrals to adult specialists familiar with MPS VI.

The transition plan also emphasized the importance of regular follow-up visits and continued multidisciplinary care. We coordinated with adult geneticists, cardiologists, orthopedists, and other specialists to ensure that the patient's medical needs were consistently addressed.

As the patient moved into adulthood, we continued to monitor for long-term complications associated with Maroteaux-Lamy syndrome. One area of particular concern was cardiac health. MPS VI can lead to progressive cardiac valve thickening and dysfunction, which may require surgical intervention. Regular echocardiograms were performed to assess cardiac function and detect any changes that might necessitate further action.

In the patient's late twenties, echocardiograms revealed significant progression of mitral and aortic valve thickening, leading to symptomatic valvular heart disease. The patient experienced fatigue, shortness of breath, and decreased exercise tolerance. After thorough evaluation by a cardiologist and cardiothoracic surgeon, it was determined that the patient required valve replacement surgery.

The patient underwent successful mitral and aortic valve replacement, which significantly improved cardiac function and quality of life. Postoperative care included cardiac rehabilitation and ongoing monitoring to ensure optimal cardiac health.

Throughout the patient's life, we remained vigilant for any new or emerging complications. Maroteaux-Lamy syndrome is a lifelong condition that requires continuous adaptation of the treatment plan to address evolving health needs. Regular follow-up visits, comprehensive assessments, and coordinated care were essential components of the patient's management strategy.

Despite the numerous challenges, the patient's journey with Maroteaux-Lamy syndrome exemplified resilience, determination, and the importance of a comprehensive, multidisciplinary approach to care. Advances in enzyme replacement therapy and surgical interventions significantly improved the patient's quality of life and extended life expectancy.

In conclusion, managing a patient with Maroteaux-Lamy syndrome is a complex and ongoing process that requires collaboration among various healthcare professionals. Early diagnosis, proactive management of complications, and coordinated care are essential to optimize outcomes and enhance the quality of life for individuals living with this rare genetic disorder. As a clinician, being part of this journey is both challenging and rewarding, offering the opportunity to make a meaningful difference in the lives of patients and their families.

❧ 23 ❧
DANBOLT-CROSS SYNDROME

I first encountered the patient during my tenure at the regional medical center. The patient presented with a myriad of symptoms that suggested a complex underlying pathology. The patient, a 32-year-old male, had been referred to me after several consultations with other specialists had failed to yield a definitive diagnosis. The patient reported a history of progressive muscle weakness, particularly in the lower limbs, which had been worsening over the past six months. Additionally, he complained of frequent falls, difficulty swallowing, and episodes of respiratory distress.

Upon initial examination, I noted the patient's emaciated appearance and apparent muscle atrophy. His gait was unsteady, and he required assistance to walk. His vital signs were within normal limits, but his respiratory rate was slightly elevated, suggesting potential respiratory muscle involvement. Neurological examination revealed diminished reflexes, muscle fasciculations, and generalized muscle weakness, more pronounced in the proximal muscles of the lower extremities.

Given the patient's presentation, my differential diagnosis included various neuromuscular disorders such as amyotrophic lateral sclerosis (ALS), myasthenia gravis, and muscular dystrophies. However, the combination of symptoms and the progressive nature of the disease suggested a possible underlying genetic disorder.

To narrow down the diagnosis, I ordered a series of tests, including electromyography (EMG) and nerve conduction studies, which revealed widespread denervation and reinnervation, consistent with a neurogenic process. Serum creatine kinase (CK) levels were mildly elevated, indicating muscle damage. Additionally, a muscle biopsy was performed, which showed evidence of chronic denervation and reinnervation, as well as scattered groups of atrophic fibers.

Given the findings, I suspected a hereditary motor neuropathy. To confirm this, I referred the patient for genetic testing, specifically looking for mutations in genes known to be associated with hereditary motor and sensory neuropathies (HMSNs). The results revealed a mutation in the gene encoding the SLC52A2 riboflavin transporter, which is indicative of Brown-Vialetto-Van Laere syndrome, also known as riboflavin transporter deficiency (RTD) type 2, a form of Danbolt-Cross syndrome.

Danbolt-Cross syndrome, or RTD, is a rare neurological disorder characterized by progressive neurodegeneration, often presenting with cranial nerve involvement, muscle weakness, and respiratory complications. It is caused by mutations in the SLC52A2 or SLC52A3 genes, which are responsible for encoding riboflavin transporters. These transporters are essential for the uptake of riboflavin (vitamin B2), a crucial component of the mitochondrial respiratory chain and cellular energy production.

The pathophysiology of Danbolt-Cross syndrome involves riboflavin deficiency at the cellular level, leading to impaired mitochondrial function and subsequent neurodegeneration. The clinical presentation can vary widely, but common features include sensorineural hearing loss, optic atrophy, bulbar palsy, and limb weakness. In severe cases, respiratory failure due to diaphragmatic paralysis can occur.

Upon confirming the diagnosis, I initiated treatment with high-dose oral riboflavin, starting at 10 mg/kg/day, divided into three doses. The rationale for this therapy is to bypass the defective transporters by providing an excess of riboflavin, thereby ensuring adequate intracellular levels to support mitochondrial function. The patient was also started on a multivitamin supplement to address any potential coexisting deficiencies.

Within the first few weeks of treatment, the patient reported a slight improvement in muscle strength and a reduction in the frequency of respiratory distress episodes. However, progress was slow, and it was evident that the neurodegenerative process had caused significant and potentially irreversible damage.

To monitor the patient's progress, I scheduled regular follow-up appointments, during which we assessed muscle strength, respiratory function, and overall neurological status. Pulmonary function tests showed a gradual improvement in forced vital capacity (FVC) and peak expiratory flow rate (PEFR), indicating a positive response to riboflavin therapy.

Despite the initial improvements, the patient's condition remained precarious. He continued to experience episodes of dysphagia and required ongoing nutritional support, including a modified diet and, at times, nasogastric tube feeding. We also initiated a pulmonary rehabilitation program to optimize respiratory muscle function and prevent further complications.

Over the course of several months, the patient's muscle strength continued to improve, albeit slowly. His gait became more stable, and he was able to walk short distances with the aid of a walker. The frequency of falls decreased, and he reported an overall improvement in his quality of life. However, the patient remained significantly disabled and required ongoing physical therapy and occupational therapy to maximize his functional abilities.

Unfortunately, despite the aggressive riboflavin therapy and supportive measures, the patient developed progressive bulbar involvement, characterized by worsening dysphagia and dysarthria. This progression highlighted the relentless nature of the neurodegenerative process in Danbolt-Cross syndrome. To address the bulbar symptoms, we consulted with a speech and swallowing therapist, who provided strategies to improve swallowing safety and communication.

As the patient's condition stabilized, we explored the possibility of genetic counseling for his family. Danbolt-Cross syndrome is inherited in an autosomal recessive manner, meaning that both parents must carry a copy of the mutated gene for their offspring to be affected. Genetic counseling would provide valuable information for the patient's family members regarding their carrier status and the risk of recurrence in future generations.

In the following year, the patient's condition remained stable with no further significant deterioration. The riboflavin therapy, combined with the multidisciplinary approach, had managed to slow the progression of the disease and improve the patient's functional abilities.

However, the patient continued to require ongoing support and rehabilitation to maintain his quality of life.

Overall, this case highlighted the importance of early diagnosis and intervention in managing rare genetic disorders such as Danbolt-Cross syndrome. The use of high-dose riboflavin therapy proved to be a pivotal component in the treatment strategy, emphasizing the role of targeted nutritional interventions in mitigating the effects of genetic deficiencies.

The patient's journey was a testament to the resilience and determination required to navigate the challenges posed by a rare neurodegenerative disorder. While the treatment did not offer a cure, it provided a means to slow the disease's progression and improve the patient's quality of life. This case underscored the critical need for ongoing research and awareness of rare genetic disorders to enhance early diagnosis, treatment, and support for affected individuals and their families.

As a medical professional, the experience of managing this case was both challenging and rewarding. It reinforced the importance of a thorough diagnostic approach, the integration of genetic testing in the diagnostic process, and the value of a multidisciplinary team in providing comprehensive care for patients with complex conditions.

In conclusion, the patient with Danbolt-Cross syndrome benefited from an early and accurate diagnosis, which allowed for the implementation of targeted riboflavin therapy. The multidisciplinary approach, including nutritional support, physical therapy, pulmonary rehabilitation, and speech therapy, played a crucial role in managing the patient's symptoms and improving his quality of life. Although the disease's progression could not be completely halted, the interventions provided a means to slow its advancement and offer the patient a better quality of life. This case serves as a reminder of the complexities and challenges inherent in managing rare genetic disorders and the importance of a holistic and patient-centered approach to care.

✺ 24 ✺
ACID SPHINGOMYELINASE DEFICIENCY

I first encountered the patient during a routine check-up. Initially, nothing seemed amiss; the patient, in their late twenties, presented with minor complaints that could easily be attributed to everyday stress and fatigue. However, as the consultation progressed, I noticed a slight yellowing of the patient's eyes and an enlarged spleen upon palpation. These signs were concerning enough to warrant further investigation.

I ordered a complete blood count, liver function tests, and an abdominal ultrasound. The blood tests revealed low platelet counts and elevated liver enzymes, while the ultrasound confirmed hepatosplenomegaly. At this stage, my differential diagnosis included various hematological and liver diseases. To narrow it down, I decided to proceed with a bone marrow biopsy and additional blood tests, including lipid panels and enzyme assays.

The bone marrow biopsy showed foam cells, which are indicative of lipid storage disorders. Foam cells are macrophages engorged with lipid-laden lysosomes, pointing towards a disorder in the metabolism of complex lipids. This finding, along with the patient's symptoms and blood work, pointed toward a lysosomal storage disease. Specifically, the combination of hepatosplenomegaly, thrombocytopenia, and foam cells led me to suspect Acid Sphingomyelinase Deficiency (ASMD), also known as Niemann-Pick Disease Types A and B.

To confirm the diagnosis, I ordered an acid sphingomyelinase enzyme activity test. This test measures the activity of the enzyme responsible for breaking down sphingomyelin, a type of lipid. In patients with ASMD, the enzyme activity is significantly reduced or absent. The results came back with markedly low enzyme activity, confirming the diagnosis of ASMD.

ASMD is a rare, inherited disorder caused by mutations in the SMPD1 gene. This gene provides instructions for making the enzyme acid sphingomyelinase, which is crucial for metabolizing sphingomyelin. The deficiency of this enzyme leads to the accumulation of sphingomyelin within cells, particularly in the liver, spleen, lungs, and bone marrow, causing the observed symptoms.

Understanding the genetic basis of ASMD, I recommended genetic counseling for the patient and their family. It was essential to identify carriers and provide them with information on the risk of passing the condition to their offspring. Genetic testing confirmed the presence of pathogenic mutations in the SMPD1 gene, solidifying our diagnosis.

The next step was to initiate a treatment plan. Unfortunately, there is no cure for ASMD, and the management is primarily supportive and symptomatic. My treatment strategy focused on addressing the specific symptoms and complications the patient was experiencing.

Given the patient's hepatosplenomegaly and thrombocytopenia, I referred them to a hematologist and a hepatologist for further evaluation and management. The hematologist recommended regular monitoring of blood counts and, if necessary, platelet transfusions to manage the thrombocytopenia. The hepatologist suggested lifestyle modifications and medications to support liver function and monitor for any signs of liver failure.

Pulmonary involvement is a common and severe complication in ASMD, particularly in Type B. Therefore, I also referred the patient to a pulmonologist for a comprehensive respiratory assessment. Pulmonary function tests revealed reduced lung capacity and interstitial lung disease. The pulmonologist prescribed bronchodilators and recommended pulmonary rehabilitation to improve the patient's breathing and overall lung function.

In addition to the specialist care, I initiated enzyme replacement therapy (ERT) with olipudase alfa, an experimental treatment aimed at replacing the deficient enzyme. While ERT is not a cure, it has shown promise in reducing the accumulation of sphingomyelin and alleviating some of the disease's symptoms. The patient was enrolled in a clinical trial, providing access to this therapy.

Monitoring the patient's progress was crucial. Regular follow-ups were scheduled to assess the effectiveness of the treatment and adjust it as needed. Blood tests, imaging studies, and pulmonary function tests were repeated at defined intervals to track the patient's condition.

Initially, the patient responded well to the treatment. The spleen size decreased slightly, and there was an improvement in platelet counts and liver enzymes. Pulmonary function tests showed stabilization of lung capacity. These positive changes indicated that the ERT was having a beneficial effect.

However, ASMD is a progressive disease, and despite

our best efforts, complications began to arise. The patient developed recurrent respiratory infections, likely due to the compromised lung function and immune system. These infections were managed with antibiotics and supportive care, but each episode took a toll on the patient's overall health.

As the disease progressed, the patient began to experience neurological symptoms, including difficulty walking and cognitive decline. These symptoms are more characteristic of Niemann-Pick Disease Type A, the more severe form of ASMD, which typically presents in infancy. However, adult patients with Type B can also exhibit neurological involvement as the disease advances.

The neurological decline prompted me to refer the patient to a neurologist for further evaluation. MRI scans of the brain revealed white matter abnormalities and atrophy, consistent with the neurodegenerative aspects of ASMD. The neurologist recommended physical therapy and occupational therapy to help maintain the patient's mobility and cognitive function for as long as possible.

Throughout this period, the patient remained under the care of a multidisciplinary team, including myself, the hematologist, hepatologist, pulmonologist, and neurologist. Our goal was to provide the best possible quality of life and manage the disease's complications as effectively as possible.

Despite the comprehensive care and experimental treatments, the patient's condition continued to deteriorate. The respiratory infections became more frequent and severe, leading to multiple hospitalizations. The patient's neurological function also declined, with worsening mobility and cognitive impairment.

In the final stages of the disease, the patient's liver function worsened significantly, leading to hepatic failure. The patient's jaundice worsened, and they developed ascites and hepatic encephalopathy, indicating advanced liver disease. The hepatologist and I discussed the possibility of a liver transplant, but the patient's overall condition and prognosis made them a poor candidate for this intervention.

The decision was made to transition the patient to palliative care, focusing on comfort and quality of life rather than aggressive treatment. Pain management, nutritional support, and psychological support were provided to the patient and their family during this difficult time.

The patient passed away peacefully, surrounded by their loved ones. The cause of death was multi-organ failure, primarily due to respiratory and hepatic complications of ASMD. This outcome, although expected given the progressive nature of the disease, was a sobering reminder of the limitations of current medical treatments for lysosomal storage disorders.

In reflecting on this case, several important points stand out. ASMD is a rare and challenging disease to diagnose and manage, requiring a multidisciplinary approach and often involving experimental therapies. The progressive nature of the disease and the involvement of multiple organ systems make it a complex and demanding condition to treat.

This case also highlights the importance of genetic counseling and testing for patients with inherited disorders. Early diagnosis and intervention can provide some benefit, but the lack of curative treatments underscores the need for ongoing research and development of new therapies.

Acid sphingomyelinase deficiency (ASMD) presents a broad spectrum of clinical manifestations due to the defective hydrolysis of sphingomyelin to ceramide and phosphorylcholine, leading to sphingomyelin accumulation in lysosomes. This lysosomal storage disrupts cellular homeostasis and function across various organs.

At the biochemical level, the absence or significant reduction of acid sphingomyelinase activity, measured through fluorometric or radiometric enzyme assays, confirms ASMD. These assays involve incubating patient-derived fibroblasts, leukocytes, or dried blood spots with synthetic sphingomyelin substrates and measuring the resultant fluorescence or radioactivity. Genetic sequencing of the SMPD1 gene complements enzyme assays by identifying pathogenic mutations, providing definitive diagnosis and insights into genotype-phenotype correlations.

The pathophysiology of ASMD involves the disruption of sphingomyelin metabolism. Sphingomyelin is a critical component of cell membranes, particularly in neuronal and hepatic cells. Its accumulation within lysosomes impairs cellular functions and triggers secondary pathological cascades, such as inflammation, oxidative stress, and apoptosis. Foam cells, laden with undigested sphingomyelin, are hallmark histological findings in ASMD, indicative of macrophage and organ-specific lipid storage.

The clinical management of ASMD is symptom-oriented, with enzyme replacement therapy (ERT) like olipudase alfa aiming to mitigate sphingomyelin accumulation. Olipudase alfa, a recombinant human acid sphingomyelinase, facilitates the breakdown of sphingomyelin, reducing lysosomal storage and associated cellular dysfunction. Clinical trials have demonstrated improvements in hepatosplenomegaly, pulmonary function, and lipid profiles, though ERT's long-term efficacy and safety are still under investigation.

Beyond ERT, hematologic support includes regular monitoring of platelet counts and potential transfusions to address thrombocytopenia. Hepatologic management involves the use of hepatoprotective agents and lifestyle modifications to support liver function. In advanced hepatic disease, liver transplantation might be considered, though its feasibility is limited by overall patient health and ASMD's multi-organ impact.

Pulmonary management focuses on mitigating interstitial lung disease and enhancing respiratory function. This involves bronchodilators, pulmonary rehabilitation, and vigilant monitoring for respiratory infections. Recurrent infections necessitate prompt antibiotic therapy and supportive care to prevent exacerbations.

Neurological involvement, particularly in advanced ASMD, is addressed through rehabilitative therapies to maintain motor and cognitive functions. MRI findings of white matter abnormalities and cerebral atrophy guide the neurological management plan. Research into targeted therapies for neurodegeneration in ASMD is ongoing, aiming to alleviate or slow disease progression.

The patient's case underscores the importance of a comprehensive, multidisciplinary approach in managing ASMD, integrating symptomatic treatments, experimental therapies, and supportive care. Genetic counseling remains crucial for patients and families, facilitating understanding of the disease's hereditary nature and implications for future generations.

In summary, ASMD's management necessitates a balance of addressing immediate symptoms, preventing complications, and participating in research initiatives to advance treatment options. This case illustrates the complexities and challenges faced in treating lysosomal storage disorders, highlighting the need for continued scientific advancements and collaborative care efforts to improve patient outcomes.

❧ 25 ❧

AARSKOG SYNDROME

When I first encountered the patient, a six-year-old male, it was during a routine pediatric checkup. His mother had brought him in, concerned about his short stature and delayed development compared to his peers. I observed his physical characteristics immediately: his height was significantly below the fifth percentile for his age, and he had a noticeable facial appearance that piqued my clinical curiosity.

Upon closer examination, I noted the following features: hypertelorism (wide-set eyes), a broad nasal bridge, and a distinctively shaped philtrum. His fingers exhibited brachydactyly, and his thumbs were broad with a slight curvature, suggestive of clinodactyly. Additionally, he had a pronounced downward slant to his palpebral fissures and a widow's peak hairline. These observations prompted me to consider a genetic syndrome.

The next step was a thorough developmental history. The patient's mother reported delays in reaching developmental milestones, particularly in motor skills. He began walking at 24 months, significantly later than the average. His speech development was also delayed; he uttered his first words around 18 months but struggled with articulation and sentence formation.

Considering the constellation of symptoms and physical features, I suspected Aarskog-Scott syndrome, a rare genetic disorder. To confirm the diagnosis, I ordered a series of tests. The most definitive was a genetic test to identify mutations in the FGD1 gene, which is associated with Aarskog syndrome. I explained to the patient's mother that while the physical examination strongly suggested this diagnosis, genetic testing was necessary for confirmation.

The genetic test was conducted using a blood sample, and it took several weeks to receive the results. Meanwhile, I referred the patient to a pediatric endocrinologist to evaluate his growth hormone levels and assess for any endocrine abnormalities that could contribute to his short stature. An X-ray of his left hand and wrist was performed to determine his bone age, which was found to be delayed by two years compared to his chronological age.

When the genetic test results returned, they confirmed my suspicion: the patient had a mutation in the FGD1 gene, solidifying the diagnosis of Aarskog syndrome. This gene mutation affects the development of facial, limb, and genital features, accounting for the patient's presentation.

The treatment plan for Aarskog syndrome is symptomatic and supportive, as there is no cure. My primary goals were to address the patient's growth delay, manage any developmental issues, and provide appropriate referrals for specialized care. Given the patient's short stature, I consulted with the pediatric endocrinologist about the potential benefits of growth hormone therapy. After evaluating the risks and benefits, we decided to initiate treatment with recombinant human growth hormone. The endocrinologist explained to the patient's mother that this treatment could help improve his growth velocity, although it would not necessarily bring his height into the normal range for his age.

In addition to growth hormone therapy, I referred the patient to a pediatric physical therapist to help with his motor skills and coordination. Early intervention in physical therapy is crucial for children with developmental delays, and I believed that a tailored program could improve his gross and fine motor skills.

Speech therapy was another critical component of his treatment plan. The patient was evaluated by a speech-language pathologist who developed a personalized therapy regimen to address his articulation issues and enhance his language development. Regular sessions were scheduled to work on his speech clarity and sentence construction.

Orthopedic consultation was necessary due to his brachydactyly and clinodactyly. The orthopedic specialist recommended observation and conservative management, as these hand abnormalities did not significantly impair his function. However, he advised regular follow-ups to monitor for any potential complications, such as joint pain or functional limitations.

Given the potential for learning disabilities in children with Aarskog syndrome, I also referred the patient to a developmental pediatrician. The developmental assessment revealed mild cognitive delays, and an individualized education program (IEP) was established in collaboration with his school to provide the necessary educational support and accommodations.

As part of comprehensive care, I also discussed genetic counseling with the patient's family. Aarskog syndrome is inherited in an X-linked recessive manner, meaning that carrier females have a 50% chance of passing the mutated gene to their offspring. The patient's mother expressed concern about the implications for future pregnancies, so I referred her to a genetic counselor to discuss family planning options and the potential risks to future children.

Over the next few years, I closely monitored the patient's progress. Regular follow-ups with the endocrinologist indicated that the growth hormone therapy was moderately successful, resulting in a noticeable increase in his growth velocity. His height, while still below average, improved significantly, and he was better able to keep up with his peers physically.

Physical and speech therapies yielded positive outcomes as well. The patient showed marked improvement in his motor coordination and speech clarity. He became more confident in social interactions and more engaged in school activities. The developmental pediatrician's ongoing support helped address his cognitive delays, and the IEP provided a structured and supportive learning environment.

Despite the many challenges, the patient's overall health remained stable. He did not experience severe complications commonly associated with Aarskog syndrome, such as cardiac or renal abnormalities, which we continuously monitored for through regular checkups and appropriate screenings.

However, it was important to remain vigilant. Aarskog syndrome can present with variable expressivity, and new symptoms or complications could arise as the patient aged. I maintained open communication with his family and other healthcare providers involved in his care, ensuring a coordinated approach to managing his condition.

By the time the patient reached adolescence, his growth had plateaued, and the decision was made to discontinue growth hormone therapy. His final adult height was below average but within a range that allowed for normal daily activities. The patient's cognitive and developmental progress continued to improve, and he achieved a level of independence appropriate for his age.

◈

Continue with
DIAGNOSIS: RARE MEDICAL CASES: VOLUME 2

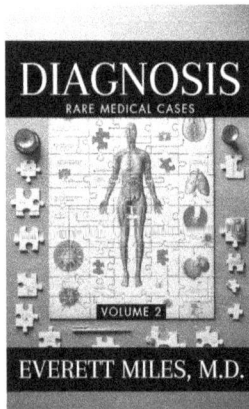

ABOUT THE AUTHOR

Dr. Everett Miles, MD, is a renowned physician with over twenty years of experience in internal medicine and diagnostics. Known for his expertise in solving complex medical cases, Dr. Miles has dedicated his career to unraveling the mysteries of rare diseases. A graduate of Johns Hopkins University School of Medicine, he combines his clinical practice with a passion for medical writing, aiming to educate and inspire both professionals and enthusiasts. Through his series, *Diagnosis: Rare Medical Cases*, Dr. Miles shares his vast knowledge and unique insights, highlighting the art and science of medicine.